REIKI

How to Increase Energy, Improve Health, and Feel Amazing With Reiki Healing

(Increase Psychic Abilities, Mind Power With Third Eye Intuition)

David Lubeck

Published by Rob Miles

David Lubeck

All Rights Reserved

Reiki: How to Increase Energy, Improve Health, and Feel Amazing With Reiki Healing (Increase Psychic Abilities, Mind Power With Third Eye Intuition)

ISBN 978-1-989990-33-9

All rights reserved. No part of this guide may be reproduced in any form without permission in writing from the publisher except in the case of brief quotations embodied in critical articles or reviews.

Legal & Disclaimer

The information contained in this book is not designed to replace or take the place of any form of medicine or professional medical advice. The information in this book has been provided for educational and entertainment purposes only.

The information contained in this book has been compiled from sources deemed reliable, and it is accurate to the best of the Author's knowledge; however, the Author cannot guarantee its accuracy and validity and cannot be held liable for any errors or omissions. Changes are periodically made to this book. You must consult your doctor or get professional medical advice before using any of the suggested remedies, techniques, or information in this book.

Upon using the information contained in this book, you agree to hold harmless the Author from and against any damages, costs, and expenses, including any legal fees potentially resulting from the application of any of the information provided by this guide. This disclaimer applies to any damages or injury caused by the use and application, whether directly or indirectly, of any advice or information presented, whether for breach of contract, tort, negligence, personal injury, criminal intent, or under any other cause of action.

You agree to accept all risks of using the information presented inside this book. You need to consult a professional medical practitioner in order to ensure you are both able and healthy enough to participate in this program.

Table of Contents

INTRODUCTION --- 1

CHAPTER 1: UNIVERSAL ENERGY IN HUMAN BODY --------- 2

CHAPTER 2: AN EXERCISE FOR YOU TO TRY -------------------- 8

CHAPTER 3: INTENT TO HEAL & SELF-TREATMENT -------- 24

CHAPTER 4: EXERCISES TO HARNESS REIKI -------------------- 31

CHAPTER 5: THE TWELVE REIKI PLACEMENTS ---------------- 37

CHAPTER 6: SELF-CARE -- 44

CHAPTER 7: REIKI SYMBOLS AND THEIR UNIQUE USES --- 61

CHAPTER 8: CHAKRAS AND REIKI -------------------------------- 75

CHAPTER 9: BALANCING THE CHAKRA FORCES -------------- 92

CHAPTER 10: FORGIVENESS LETTER ----------------------------- 99

CHAPTER 11: REIKI AND RELATED CONCEPTS -------------- 110

CHAPTER 12: TWENTY-FOUR HAND POSITIONS IN REIKI 122

CHAPTER 13: OPTIMIZING THE BENEFITS OF REIKI HEALING --- 132

CHAPTER 14: TIPS -- 135

CHAPTER 15: WHAT IS REIKI? ----------------------------------- 140

CHAPTER 16: BENEFITS AND LIMITATIONS OF REIKI ----- 147

CHAPTER 17: TOOLS FOR TESTING YOUR ENERGY -------- 160

CHAPTER 18: UNIVERSAL RADIATION, UNDERSTANDING THE AURA -- 174

CHAPTER 19: EXTRA REIKI TIPS---- ERROR! BOOKMARK NOT DEFINED.

CONCLUSION -- 191

Introduction

Reiki cannot be learned through books, brochures, videos, or audiotapes. To become a practitioner, it is necessary to receive, personally, the initiation (tuning) by a teacher properly trained for it. Upon initiation, this book can become a guide for the new practitioner; however, in no way can it be considered as a self-learning manual.

Whoever is willing to practice it without proper initiation will not be using Reiki energy and will be compromising his own energy with harmful results for his health. To use the Reiki technique, it is essential to find a trained teacher first.

There are plenty of books on this subject on the market, so thanks again for choosing this one! Every effort was made to ensure it is full of as much useful information as possible. Please enjoy!

Chapter 1: Universal Energy In Human Body

The force of life is a subtle energy that flows and surrounds routes, such as chakras and meridians, and it is ever present in all living beings. The vital force nourishes and encourages the functioning of all cells of the body. If your life force is low, you will probably feel brittle. You're likely to be sick. Enhancing your strength in life will help your body heal and remain healthy. Your life force flow becomes disrupted, causing your body organs to function diminished. If you have adverse ideas or adverse emotions about yourself, your general body balance (mental, emotional and physical) will be troubled, then you get sick. Thoughts and emotions have an immense impact on life force.

It is the inspiration for our whole existence. In truth, the warm temperature of the sun that heats our bodies, the gasoline that we use in our car, the power used inside the household, is the same energy forms. It sustains life and provides vital energy to all living systems. At the most fundamental level, starting from the stars to as small as atoms, the Universal Energy is present in everything we see and do.

Sensitive To The Atmospheric Energy

Our souls can feel the universal vibrations been more aware of the energy present around. They tend to sense the power of the surroundings and even that of people who aren't associated with them. Because the planet's vibration keeps increasing, more individuals are becoming receptive to the regular strength that surrounds us. Right here are seven indications that you are an amazing delicate empath for the Universal Energy:

Sensitive To Other Humans' Feelings

Empaths can often assume what another individual feels, and they can even perceive their feelings as though they were theirs. They can also tell you what someone else feels, even if that person isn't there with them.

This can be arduous, which is why protecting their power is very essential to an empath. There are plenty of signs of survival for empaths and extremely sensitive people to help prevent and alleviate an emotional overload.

Feeling Uncomfortable In Enclosed Spaces Or Crowded Areas

Empaths might also be overwhelmed and probably barely agitated while in a crowded space or even in some public locations. This is because the human beings around them are connected to them and there is an inflow of energy.

The development of protective tool for the sake of protecting the interest of sensitive people who are more aware about their environment which suggests that certain sounds, lights and smell could make them feel better.

A Very Good Intuition

Since empathy is so aware of the setting and other people's energy, their instinct is often very powerful. Before an event happens they can comprehend it and can experience when someone they care about is going through a difficult moment.

Looking For Spiritual Connection

People who are more sensitive to the Universal Energy have a profound desire to find a spiritual link with their partner, establish their spiritual family, or even a home with which they can resonate profoundly on a deep psychological level.

Strong Desires

Empaths have very vibrant and excessive objectives, complete of creativity that they often maintain in mind. A chance to visit other places is a dream come true for such individuals to explore other levels of reality.

Experience Growth In Their Inner Self

Empaths are prepared to open their minds at any time to see the world from many angles because of their empathy, creativity, and a willingness to learn more about their soul's requirements.

Via different reports along with gaining access to kundalini electricity or opening the third eye, they regularly experience spiritual awakenings.

Non-Stop Search Of The Reason For Existence

Jobs, families, material security, or seeking pleasure is not all there is to life for empaths. They have the feeling that life is something much bigger and deeper. This feeling prompts them to think of life's true meaning.

Empaths attempt to incorporate themselves and create their private contributions in a consistent and beneficial manner into the planet. Since this strategy can become their life's symbolic value, they may sometimes feel disgusted by someone who does not share this perspective.

To Develop & Nurture Your Sensitivity to the Universal Energy

Examine and evaluate the various seasons of the year and the lunar stages of your mental states.

Have a paper and write down your most vivid dreams and make sure you're perusing it regularly.

Attempt to discover patterns that are showing up regularly. This will assist you to interpret and discover a deeper significance in your dreams.

Mediate more to feel the power of all living humans, particularly in nature, and how things are interconnected.

Observing the sky and star-looking practice deepens your link to the world.

Chapter 2: An Exercise For You To Try

So when you've got a spare minute then, perhaps tonight in bed, really do have a proper go at this exercise.

Take yourself back to the beginning of the universe again and try to feel what it was like. We say feel rather than think, because trying to use your head to figure all this out, won't work at all.

Logic is not going to be of much help to you on this journey.

Feelings are the name of the game here.

Really reach out with your feelings. Ask yourself what would there be at the beginning of time and wait for your feelings - your intuition - that still small voice inside of you, to answer.

Or ask yourself what it would be like to be dead for all eternity, and again wait for your feelings or intuition to answer.

If nothing comes up for you, in terms of answers, don't worry. It's the knowing that some part of you is always there that's the important bit.

The understanding that you cannot - not be.

The knowing that no matter what happens you, as a consciousness, are immortal.

An extraordinary thought

Really play with this thought, this idea that you've always been here.

That there's never been a 'time' - when you were not here!

Indeed, dare to think the thought, dare to feel the feeling that...

Long, long ago in a time before time, there existed an extraordinarily powerful energy which began speculating about who and what it was.

And that extraordinarily powerful energy was...

YOU

Wow, how does that make you feel?

Well, if you've already done the exercise we suggested, your feelings may be that - hmmm, you know something, this may just possibly, be possible.

Now, just hold onto this possibility for a moment, and...

...we hope you've brought your umbrella with you because yes, that's correct.

We are suggesting that...

YOU are ALL THAT IS...

The Supreme Being, Infinite Consciousness, God, Goddess, All That Is or any other name you choose to give it.

Now, before you throw up your arms in horror and disgust at this suggestion – just try allowing the possibility...

moment and allow your feelings, not your head, to come to the fore.

Right oh then.

Please take a break now and consider what has been said. Go and do the exercise we've just suggested, if you haven't already done it, then come back and we'll continue.

Go on now – off you go.

You're not going to miss anything. We won't go any further until you come back – we promise.

We'll just wait right here.

Okay you're back, so did you do it? Did you?

Only you know the answer to that one.

But we'll give you the benefit of the doubt, should we? And accept that you really, really did or really, really meant to, or really, really will or would have, if only you had had the time, the energy, the patience, the…

……………………….… (You can fill in the blank with your very own really, real excuse).

If you did do the exercise, great, if you didn't that's okay too.

Just remember, though, that the more you put into this book the more you'll get out of it.

Anyway let's carry on regardless.

We left you with the thought, the feeling, that the extraordinarily powerful energy source – All That Is – could actually be you. Now some of you may have had a little trouble with that, and some may be having trouble in believing in the concept of there being an All That Is, any All That Is, at all.

So let's delve a little more deeply into this subject right now.

This is, of course, only for those people who cannot yet accept that...

THEY are - All That Is.

Belief in God, Goddess, All That Is

Belief in God, Goddess, All That Is, Supreme Being - or any other name you wish to attach to this possibility...

...has had some real bad press just recently, so it's understandable if people are having a problem with it.

People, quite rightly, question the existence of a Supreme Being, a God, who can let all the atrocities that occur in the world, take place.

Why, they say, if there is such a thing as a Supreme Being would it let all these things happen?

How could a being so immensely powerful, who is supposed to be so compassionate and loving, allow people to starve to death? Why would it allow all these wars to take place?

Why would it permit anything bad to happen to anyone?

Surely if there is a Supreme Being, it must be powerful enough to fix all these things at a stroke, mustn't it?

So, you reason, if there is a Supreme Being and it is powerful enough to fix all these things, as it should be if it is a All That Is, and it doesn't, it can only mean one of two things...

Two choices

1. There is a Supreme Being but it doesn't really care enough about us to help.

Or

2. There is no Supreme Being at all.

Now if statement number 1 is true, we have a couple of ways in which we can proceed. We can try to figure out a way to get it to like and love us or we can say – "Why should we take any notice of a Supreme Being who doesn't love us and won't take care of us"?

And just ignore the whole subject altogether.

The path of ignorance

Many, many people have chosen this latter path. The path of ignore-ance.

But how can this prevailing attitude be changed?

How can anyone be encouraged to choose the possibility of All That Is, over the comfort of ignorance?

Well, by raising the consciousness of people to another level.

And how do we do this?

Yes, you guessed it, through Reiki, of course.

But before we get onto that subject, let's examine what happens to the people who want to figure out how to get All That Is to love and care for them.

People wanting to discover the way to this kind of reality usually follow the directions given in some kind of organised religion.

It doesn't really matter which particular one is followed, and quite often their family has already chosen it for them anyway. All religions are attempting to lead their followers in a similar direction.

And all are useful - until they are not, and that's when the trouble starts.

The Laws of God

Religions require strict adherence to the rules and regulations as set out by the founder of their particular religion.

Most purporting to having received these rules directly from whatever it is they call God, Goddess, All That Is.

With the implication from all being – you won't receive the love and care of All That Is unless you abide by our rules, which they have now imperiously called 'The Laws of God'.

Now what people seem to forget when they are being guided by these religions is that they're often many hundreds of years old.

The rules and regulations, sorry 'Laws of God', were made in times when the people weren't quite as sophisticated as they are today.

They were in abject fear and awe of their religious leaders.

But that is no longer the case in some countries today. Some of these people are beginning to ask questions of their religion.

Do not question the wisdom of All That Is

True Believers would say, we must not question the wisdom of All That Is, because All That Is works in mysterious ways.

But for some people - people in hardship and pain - people suffering from the most horrendous atrocities - people watching their children die because of religious wars or for the want of a little food and some clean water...

...this answer doesn't come anywhere near to being enough.

So the True Believers change tack a little.

They then tell us that the suffering we are experiencing will make us better people.

They say it is like making a better quality of steel. The more heat and the more hammering it takes, the stronger and purer, it will be.

And this, they say, is what is actually happening and that we should bear with it.

If this still does not pacify us, True Believers tell us that because of our massive suffering we must be special people and will get tremendous rewards in heaven.

People begin to doubt their religion

Now with all of this going on, is it not surprising that people begin to doubt their religion?

Well, fortunately, they do but, unfortunately, they also begin to doubt in any Supreme Being at all.

When things are at their darkest and you cry out for help.

When you've taken so much - and you can't take anymore...

You know that All That Is has been watching.

You know The Supreme Being has seen your suffering.

Seen this hardship and pain that you have endured.

You know it knows this is more than any one person should ever be allowed to bear.

Trusting in All That Is

You desperately want to trust in All That Is. You want to believe that it will only allow so much suffering to happen to you, and then mercifully, make it stop.

You know this is how it's supposed to work.

But the pain and the suffering continue.

All That Is does not answer your prayers. You cry and beseech. You pray harder and implore. You make threats and then beg for forgiveness. You promise you'll be good from now on.

You try to make bargains you know you'll never keep.

You try everything you can, until finally, you get so angry and disillusioned that...

...You stop believing altogether

It's much easier to say you don't believe. You find out that there are thousands, indeed, millions of people who don't believe.

In fact it's quite cool not to believe.

You wonder at how you could have been so foolish to have been taken in by all this nonsense in the first place.

A Supreme Being that looks after us - how ridiculous!

It somehow makes you feel better, now that you've seen through the hoax.

Things might not actually be any better, but at least you've found out the truth.

And this is a scenario which takes place on a daily basis around the world, and has done so for many, many years.

It'll probably carry on for many, many more years too.

The True Believers would have it that everything has just been a test of your faith. And the fact that you have lost this faith is proof that you are not worthy - are somehow inferior because you weakened.

Which, of course, is a favourite ploy.

For you see, making you feel unworthy and inferior makes them feel ever so much more worthy and superior.

At this late stage, however, it cuts no ice, and you continue to say you disbelieve. Except, against all the odds, a part of you, maybe a very small part of you, has still not given up completely.

It won't be denied; it somehow knows better.

Out of touch religions

This is the experience of too many people. Too many people have been let down. And the clichés and platitudes that trip easily from the tongues of these out of touch religious leaders do not help.

People don't want to hear that they will get their rewards in heaven.

They don't want to hear that life is supposed to be a school full of hardship and pain...

...a place where you come solely to learn how to bear suffering because it will somehow make you a better person!

To the people of today these things no longer make any sense.

And to these people who have had this kind of experience with their religion, we offer the following words of hope.

All religions are entirely man made.

They do not represent the word of All That Is in any way shape or form.

The rules and regulations they adhere to are simply that – rules and regulations – they are not 'Laws of God' – they were just made up by man.

If you are still involved with a religion and it works for you, then that's great.

We have no problem with that.

As we have already said, all religions are useful until they are not, and what we mean by that is this...

...Religions are okay when first starting out

Religions offer a well-trodden path for you to follow.

They're perfect for when you are just starting out and need to know what to do, when to do it and who to turn to for advice if it is needed.

They're kind of like a paint-by-numbers picture.

If you stay within the marked lines they allow you to create a passable painting, whilst not being too demanding. And you also get to practice some of the more elementary techniques in a very safe environment.

The problem is, of course, you can only end up with the picture that they have carefully outlined for you. You cannot use your own free will to be wonderfully and spontaneously creative.

Now if you are quite happy to be a paint-by-numbers artist this approach is absolutely fine.

If you want to be a great artist in your own right, however, you might find it a bit limiting.

And this, you will discover, holds true for all religions as well.

Moving beyond religion

Once you have reached this point, the point when you begin to realise that there must be something more. Wouldn't it be nice if the religion, and the religious leaders themselves, said to you...

..."Well done. You've come as far as we can take you. It's now time to walk your own path for we don't wish to limit your growth. The guidance you require for your next steps will come from within you.

You must now learn to meditate and follow your own counsel. And don't worry; we'll always be here to help if you need us."

Wouldn't that be nice?

Wouldn't it be nice for a religion to be honest enough with you to say these things? To actively promote and support your individual emergence as a powerful spiritual being in your own right.

But they don't, and they won't.

Why?

Because religion is, unfortunately, very big business.

The machinery behind these religions is vast and very expensive.

The amount of people earning their livings from these religions is vast. The power, prestige and social standing awarded to these people is vast too.

And they're not about to give any of this up without a fight.

Without you, they are out of business.

Chapter 3: Intent To Heal & Self-Treatment

Now that you are attuned and you know the principles you are ready to start healing. The intent to heal is truly as simple as laying your hands on yourself or another person and urging with little effort the Reiki to flow, however a small ritual of hand placement can make things go faster in the beginning. There are many who feel when they being a treatment with intent to heal that asking the energy out loud to flow is the best way to get the energy to respond quickly. Showing proper respect and honoring the energy is a good habit to get into, coupling that respect with the intent to heal hand positions will allow the energy to come faster and stronger.

Intent to heal hand positions:

The first position you can use for intent to heal on yourself or others involves bringing your hands into the position of namaste before you begin the healing.

With your hands still in this position you will place them above the heart, giving a bow of your head in respect and then quietly ask the Reiki to begin to move through you.

The second position involves placing your hands above you're had with your palms upward and showing to the sky. From here you will picture the Reiki is moving down from the sky and into your palms and then farther into your body hitting all of your chakra's as it goes.

These are the two beginning hand positions for Reiki healing, they get everything started and it is important (as noted on on the checklist in the previous chapter) to always remember to do one of them before you begin a healing. There is no elaborate ceremony needed for Reiki healing just these simple hand gestures and asking the help of the energy is generally all that is needed. If you have the permission of someone to heal them and you wish to do so, that is all the true intent to heal that you need.

When you go into a healing and allow the energy to come, remember the word surrender. When you surrender or give into Reiki you are merely allowing it to flow through you and allowing the energy itself to guide you. You will not try to guide the energy because the Reiki itself truly knows better and will show you exactly what needs to be focused on. You should remain aware and don't become lax in attention when you surrender because the Reiki will show you a path to follow and you need to stay aware of that so you or the person you are healing can get the best energy and healing possible. You have to be willing and have a great deal of trust in the energy itself, be sure it will guide you in the right direction.

Self-treatment

Treating yourself is one of the most important parts of Reiki especially for a beginner. This should be done daily when you are first starting out. One big reason for self healing is that it allows you to become more attuned and familiar with Reiki on your own schedule. The other reason you should practice on yourself daily is to ensure that you are open, receptive and prepared to pass Reiki on to others if you plan to heal anyone else. By improving your own health, you will be able to balance easier and find a true center quickly and finally, it allows you to become more aware of what the energy is trying to tell you and where to focus. Like with many things in life the more you do it the better you get at it.

The basic hand positions for self healing:

Link your hands together on the top of your head

Place one hand on your forehead, then place the other at the back of your neck about one hand length above the base of your neck.

Place your hands gently over your eyes

Place your hands gently over your ears

Place one hand on your upper torso and place the other on your rib cage.

Place your hands on your hips

When you are beginning the process of self healing it is good to first go through each hand position so you can get comfortable with them. Just move your hands through the motions and relax your body in each position for up to 5 minutes. As you practice you will want to continue to picture your energy, go through this practice process as many times as you need until you begin to feel confident that you know them. Once you have confidence in knowing the positions start to open your mind and listen to intuition, let it guide you to where your hands should go next and how long they should stay in any one position trusting your inner guide is one of the most important things you can do for Reiki healing. The good thing to remember in Reiki is that there is really no such thing as a wrong move or a mistake, you can do no harm with Reiki. When you heal the divine deity will always be watching you and guiding you to the right positions and places ensuring a successful healing. Gradually let your hands be guided by your intuition. As you practice and have a little patience you will gain experience and begin to trust your inner guidance. You cannot really make a mistake. Your healing sessions are always watched over by the Divine to ensure that your efforts will always be rewarded.

Once you are comfortable with the hand positions you can begin your first self treatment. You will begin by showing respect and honor to the Reiki energy and the Divine. You will use one of the intent to heal hand positions and carefully call upon the energy, if you feel the need for extra assistance you can call out to your Reiki guides or Angels to assist you. We always have more than one presence watching and guiding us throughout our treatment.

Once you have begun with the proper respect and hand position you will listen for that guidance and allow your hands to move to the needed points and memorized positions. Sometimes you will find that you go through all of the positions and others you may only go through one or two, it all depends on which chakra and area needs help to make the energy flow during a given session. Time is another factor that can change from healing to healing, trust your instinct on how long you must keep your hands laid in any position. There is no right or wrong dedicated time frame to energy healing.

Using your intuition and focus once you feel that enough time has passed for healing, you will again pay respect to the Divine and the Reiki energy and allow it to go back to a normal flow around you. That is all that is needed for self healing. It may seem simplistic, but when dealing with powerful life energy like this you don't need to place it in a fancy package and the more you self heal the stronger your feeling and connection to the energy will be.

Chapter 4: Exercises To Harness Reiki

There are many exercises which you can perform to harness reiki and they are really easy to do. You can make others learn about it as well as recharge yourself with the healing power of it of mental and physical level. Here are some of the awesome quick exercises which you can practice on your own and feel relaxed.

16. The Breathing Exercise

Make sure to sit at a quiet place and make yourself comfortable. Now lie back or sit somewhere and then close your eyes. Make sure you do not have any disturbing thing around you such as cellphone or TV which can distract you. Now concentrate on your breathing. Next, put your hands on your lap and now breathe slowly by exhaling or inhaling. Imagine yourself with connecting with the universal life energy which flows the energy in your body.

Keep on doing that for about five minutes and you will see how easy you will feel. It is important for you to practice this exercise every day because it makes you feel easy and fresh. You feel stronger inside and the feeling of blood flowing inside you will make you feel better. Now open the eyes really slow and then stretch yourself so you can come back to the consciousness. This way you will feel calmer and more focused towards the important things of your life.

17. Clean the surrounding

Make sure to keep your surroundings clean. It is important to keep the room clean from all the clothes and books scattered. The surroundings show the state of your mind and if the room is clean and lighter on the things, you will see that you will be able to sleep properly as well. So before lying down today, make sure to take out 10 minutes and keep the things on their places.

18. The Objects

The objects and the things which are in your room or your surrounding have an impact on your thinking. If you have something light colored or dark colored around you even that has an impact on your brain. If you keep the essential oils in your room and the fragrance spreads all around, it makes you feel easy and you will be able to sleep better. The next day when you wake up, you will feel better on the brain and your mood will be happier as well. So the things around you matter, make sure to have those which have a good impact on you and your personality.

19. The food intakes

Make sure to take the healthy food and avoid any kind of fast foods. When we go outside, we tend to see every fast food and get attracted to it. Do not make it a habit but instead have fruits and nutrients food which benefit you in a longer run. Food helps you to maintain the energy and keeps you fit also. If you do not in take the right food, it will affect your body negatively and you will be in a depressing mood. Food gives you the nutrients which you need in order to sustain all day long which is why people tend to take the proper meals of three times a day and exercise as well so that it can digest better and does not irritate their digestive system.

20. Quick Picks

You can do some of the things quickly as an exercise which won't even take 10 minutes of your life but you will actually start feeling better. Whether you are in office or at school, try this in your break and you will be back up with the energy level which you were in the morning. So, find a place to sit where it is comfortable. Make sure to put one hand on your forehead and then other on the stomach. Now drift both hands gently the opposite sides and keep on doing that for 10 minutes. This will ease up both the main points of stress and you will see that you will be active for the rest of the day.

21. The Aid of Sleep

If you have a hard time sleeping at night then this is the best exercise which you can try and you will surely experience that you will get a good night sleep. Even if you get 2 hours of sleep at night, it will feel like you have taken full 8 hours of sleep. Make sure you have eaten well and then before sleeping, do this exercise. Lie back and relax. Now place one hand on the forehead and other on the stomach. Now breathe in and out slowly and keep on rubbing your forehead. You will feel relaxed on your body. Do this for about 5 minutes but very slowly.

This will help you get a better sleep at night and you will no longer need to be up being irritated that you could not even sleep.

22. The Principles

There are certain principles which you can learn in order to meditate with Reiki by your own. The more you know about them the more easily it will get. It keeps your heart calm and you will be good to go for the week. Place your hand on the heart and repeat these sentences to yourself such as work hard, do not be worried, be grateful, be kind to others, do not be irate and more just like these. These will help you retain the energy and you will feel motivated by reminding yourself of these principles. If you memorize them, it will get easier for you do it anytime you feel stressed. And it will become your habit, which means that you will not stress on small things anymore.

Chapter 5: The Twelve Reiki Placements

Since your aim is to direct ki to different parts of your body with your hands, you will need to know how to hold them and where to place them. While advanced practitioners make use of various hand gestures and go all over the body, self-treatment focuses on twelve body parts and makes use of only one hand gesture.

Hold your hands away from you palms outward, as if saying "stop" or as if pushing something away from you. Now place your fingers and thumbs together so there's no gap between them. And bingo! Except for position five, that's the only hand gesture you will use for yourself throughout the twelve placements.

Close your eyes and take several deep breaths. As you breathe in, understand that you are drawing ki into yourself. Now raise your hands, knowing that they will direct the ki to wherever you place them. That ki will come out of your palms and infuse whatever you touch with universal life energy.

At each spot, inhale deeply to invoke the ki, then exhale slowly to help increase its flow. How long you spend on each spot depends on you, which is why a session can last anywhere from 10 to 40 minutes.

Normally, you should spend the same amount of time in each position. But if you have some health issue or if some spot seems to require more attention, then it's alright to spend more time on it. This bit has to be addressed.

Those who have been practicing reiki regularly claim that no two sessions are ever alike. Due to changing circumstances, practitioners (and even novices, sometimes) feel a sort of "pull" toward a certain spot. It can range anywhere from an unconscious skipping of a body part, to a compunction to spend more time on another. This is the result of a higher power directing them to address some imbalance they may not even be aware of.

Done regularly, the following exercise not only improves your ability to conduct ki, it also increases your sensitivity to a higher, guiding power.

Place your palms lightly on your face to either side of your nose. The tips of your fingers and thumbs should face upward, so that your palms cover both your eyes.

It's believed that this heals headaches, toothaches, hay fever, sinus blockages, eye problems, and balances the pituitary gland.

Place your palms above your ears on either side of your head, then bend your fingers so that the tips of your middle and ring fingers meet on the crown of your head.

This cures headaches, improves blood pressure and one's sense of balance, as well as provides mental clarity and insight.

Move your palms to the back of your head. Your left hand should rest in a lower position, such that your left palm rests on the fleshy part above your neck but below your skull. Your right hand should be in the higher position so that your palm rests against the back of your skull. Your right thumb should rest lightly against your left pinky finger.

This helps with sleeping disorders and stress. It's also believed to help release past hurts and frustrations.

Move your palms forward to cup your cheeks. Your wrists should touch below your chin, your thumbs should rest against your lower jaw, while your index fingers should rest below your tragi (the slightly hard part of your outer ear that sort of covers the ear hole). With all your other fingers kept together, everything else should fall into place.

This treats metabolic disorders, sore throat, tonsillitis, flu, hoarseness, the vocal cords, lymph nodes, as well as the thyroid and parathyroid glands.

Place your right hand against your neck and make a V with your thumb on one side and your fingers on the other. Your right thumb should rest below your right jaw, while your right fingers should lightly grasp the left side of your neck. You want the palm of your right hand to rest very gently against your throat. If you're a man, your Adam's apple should rest lightly in the hollow of your right palm.

Lower your left hand and place your left palm against the bony part of your upper chest—your collarbone, some two to three inches above your solar plexus. The lower part of your right wrist should rest gently above and cover the upper fingers of your left hand.

This also treats the thyroid and parathyroid glands, lymph nodes, vocal chords, and larynx.

Lower your hands and place your index fingers and thumbs beneath your chest, such that the tips of your middle fingers meet over your solar plexus.

This treats the heart, lungs, thymus gland, and respiratory system.

Rest your palms on your stomach, just above your navel. Your fingers should point downward a little, so that the tips of your middle and index fingers meet.

This promotes digestion, treats the spleen, pancreas, liver, gall bladder, and promotes emotional well-being.

Keeping your fingers in their exact same position (pointing downward slightly so that the tips of your index and middle fingers meet), lower your hands so your palms rest against your pelvic bones and your fingers meet just above your groin area.

This treats the abdominal organs, bladder, urethra, intestines, appendix, and reproductive organs. It also treats menstrual, menopausal, and digestive disorders.

Lift your hands over your shoulders and gently rest the tips of your fingers and thumbs on your shoulder blades. If you're flexible enough, try to rest the palms of your hands on your shoulders. Your hands should not touch each other, but remain a few inches apart.

This also treats the thyroid and parathyroid glands, as well as the vocal cords, larynx, and lymph nodes. It's also believed to heal emotional issues like guilt.

Bring your hands down on either side of you and rest your palms on your mid-back. The tips of your fingers should not touch, but should rest lightly on either side of your spine two to three inches below your shoulders opposite the upper half of your stomach.

This treats respiratory problems and promotes a healthy heart, as well as any emotional issues you might have.

Rest your palms against your lower back, an inch or two above your buttocks. Your fingers should again point downward slightly, such that the tips of your ring fingers touch just above your sacrum (the triangular bone in your lower back).

This treats the digestive tract, as well as repressed emotions.

Lower your hands further against your sacrum. This time, your hands will form a downward pointing triangle, such that your ring and pinky fingers meet at their tips.

This treats the same issues cited for position eight.

Chapter 6: Self-Care

Everyone wants to lead a good life. It is everyone's wish to live a healthy and cheerful lifestyle, and id this could be bought, then no one would be living any kind of life that they don't feel comfortable with. It is everyone's responsibility to offer themselves the kind of life they need. You have all it takes to make yourself happy and free from stress and worries. You want to be happy; you want to a respectable person, and you want everyone around you to look at you and say, "this is the kind of life I want to live because it is exactly what I deserve."
Don't wait for anyone to do this for you. Go for everything it takes to make yourself the kind of people you always admire.

You have the assignment of taking good care of yourself in a way that you find better. You need to look good and admirable. Someone sees you as a role model, and they wish to become exactly like you. Take this task and maintain what they see from you that make them wish to be you. Aim at making yourself look better than that and keep motivating them to believe that they truly deserve this kind of life and should start following your steps to become like you.

You need to treat yourself in a way that makes everyone want to take lessons on what they need to do to feel better, to look healthy, and to remain happy always. Taking good care of yourself will give those who are looking up to you a reason to focus on what they want to grow into and will influence them to love the way you are living your life and handling every situation of it.

Your Wellbeing

Self-care needs a huge sense of wellbeing. This is yet another task that is added to your duties. Just when you thought that someone somewhere is responsible for your wellbeing and should work super hard to keep you happy and maintain your good living standard for you, then boom, you are wrong! This is your duty, it is automatically assigned for you, and you don't need anyone to remind you to do this.

It is your responsibility to ensure that you record good health status, you are mentally stable, and your emotions are well balanced. This is the only way you can like the kind of lifestyle you are giving yourself and feel happy about it. You have to make yourself proud of yourself and contented with your level of life.

Your Wellbeing Domains

There are key tools that everyone requires for their personal wellbeing. These are a tool, and so they have to be well maintained. Just like a machine, when any part breaks down, it becomes useless until it is repaired and its good condition maintained. Your wellbeing domains also have to be recognized and well taken care of for you to be the better person that you deserve.

The first and the most important domain for your well-being is a healthy, well-balanced diet. You need to grow and not just grow. You need to grow healthy and attractive. This is the number one thing that will make you feel happy about yourself. You will look at yourself and say, "damn, I am proud of who I am." This feeling keeps you motivated to work hard to maintain this picture if yourself.

Secondly, you need to have a good mind control tactics. Put yourself in a position to think positively about every situation and respond calmly to every reaction. Don't let yourself get hurt at the site of everything that happens to you. If everything around you affects you negatively, then you are going to lose it. Take good care of yourself by taking care of your thoughts because you are not a slave and you have all the rights and, most importantly the ability to make yourself remain healthy.

My Current Wellbeing

Your current wellbeing is determined by how you lived your past life. What you offered yourself and the kind of activities you allowed yourself to engage in is very important in this case. When you lived negatively in the past, then you are more likely to experience a tough time in the present. You will be left thinking of the negative things that happened in the past, and this will keep your mind stuck in one place, hindering you from moving on to a better life.

To make yourself comfortable with the current situation, you have to stop thinking of the past and the things that had already happened, whether good or bad. This is the only thing that can set your mind free and unoccupied, giving it another chance to start afresh and make you a happy person. You deserve a better life so don't be a slave of the past. Let go and move on with a different focus and target.

My Future Wellbeing

The state of life that you will be in some time to come should not be anything close to your current condition. Your future should be great, so work towards making it great. Your future well-being starts now. The way you are living your life currently and the activities you are involved with will tell where you will be in the future so don't tie yourself to anything unhealthy if you want a better future.

Start now, and build a healthy future just for you. The love that you offer to others should first be offered to you by none other than you. Be this person that you expect to make you happy. The person that you think is responsible for your wellbeing is not your parent, your sibling, your child or your spouse. This person is you. Accept the task today and build the future of your desire.

Never sit back and relax, thinking that in the future, you will become a better person than who you are today. This is the only best time for you to make a change. Start today and aim higher. Focus on giving yourself something that you never had before, something that will make you happy for the rest of your life. Do something that is worth your effort and that you'll sit down someday to look back and smile for the kind of achievement that comes with it.

Aspiration for Balance

You really need to balance between the things that you do. The feeling that keeps motivating you to work hard is the same feeling that should motivate you to make good use of your life. Be eager to live the best lifestyle. A good lifestyle is well balanced between activities and normal life. Learn how to grow yourself. Know how to balance work, exercise, family, and the time you spend with yourself.

Spending time with yourself means you think about no one else or anything else but only you. You are alone, and the only thing that is in your inner world at this moment is only you. All the attention you focus on yourself and allow your mind to be stress-free. Don't think about the things that make you worried. Only think about yourself, interview yourself and answer the questions that come along personally and honestly.

The wrongs that you had committed in the past should aspire you to doing something better than what you did back then that will balance your thoughts and emotions, giving you the courage o push hard towards a great future. You can go out for a walk or engage in any activity that will refresh your mind and give room for new ideas that can make your future better.

My Wellbeing Plan Step by Step

Having a good plan for yourself is a good idea. For you to live the kind of life you deserve, it is important to have a well-structured plan that will lead to your wellbeing. You need to reorganize yourself to create room for every good thing. Schedule yourself well and master when you need to do what and where forehead duration. This will always keep you on toes and make you do everything at the right time and place.

You will never have difficulty working on your wellbeing when you have a good plan for your activities. Develop a timetable for yourself that involves everything you need to stay better. Only do what should be done at any time and don't s spend even the slightest moment of your time doing what should not be done at that time. This will give you an easy time managing yourself and focusing on important things only. You will live a happy life that is stable and free from distractions.

Tackling Skills

Some skills can be applied in trying to maintain your wellbeing. Have a picture of yourself and view every activity that you participate in. What is the influence of every activity in your wellbeing? What is influencing you negatively, and what is bringing progress to your life? When you notice something that is dragging you behind, think of how best you can handle it to bring a positive change in your life.

Anything that is not making you happy should be dropped and focus on things that make you feel important and fit to engage in other activities. Find a better and the most effective way of handling things that delay your progress or impact negatively towards your wellbeing. Handle everything carefully and never be afraid of losing to the opponent. When something is trying to pull you down, face it confidently, and take the unobvious direction to challenge it and win the battle.

You should not be afraid of trying something new. Go for what you think can bring healthy change to your mind. Welcome the right state of emotions that will help you developmentally, emotionally, spiritually, and also physically.

Daily Activity

The kind of activities you engage in from day to day should contribute to your wellbeing. If any activity does not impact genuinely to your wellbeing, then there's no need holding on to it. Focus your attention on something that makes you feel healthy. Something that protects your self-worth and makes others see you as a person they would also want to be.

You should engage yourself in sports activities to allow your mind to relax and be attentive and for your body to be flexible and ready for anything that comes along. Your mind should be free from anger and hatred. These are things that only bring pain and suffering to your heart and your mind that you can never think of anything apart from causing troubles.

Your daily activities show be the kind that makes you feel relaxed and ready to face what is to come next. They should free your mind from negative thoughts that lead you to the wrong direction and decisions. This will allow you to love yourself even better because you will only think about their positive side.

Creative Self-Care

Something creative is something unique. Developing unique ideas that you can apply to make yourself feel better to bring the best and unique changes to our lives. Creativity leads in the best direction, and you are left thinking of what you have done as the best option ever and that there is no other person that can beat you in making yourself happy.

You will have no one to look up for in order to be healthy and presentable. You will let go of all the doubt and fear that make you stick to one point and fix your mind in a single idea that is not even helping you to grow. You should have the best and unique strategies that help your mind to expand and relate to everything that makes you healthy and physically fit.

Listening to Your Emotions

Emotions are the dictators of your movement. Pay attention to what your emotions want. How they make you feel is very important as it helps you identify your areas of weakness and enable you to work towards strengthening your weakest points. When you carefully listen to your emotions, you will be gain a lot of information about what you need and what you don't need.

Listening to your emotions does not restrict you from doing only what your emotions tell you to do. You have all the power to change your thoughts and go for what suits you better than the other. Make a decision depending on what you want and the world's view towards it. For you to move on, or for anyone to progress well, you should feel free to go against most emotions that make you feel bad because it is toxic to your health and even your relationship with those around you.

Tackling Toolkit

Here comes the button that you have to press to open the way for new and great opportunities to help you learn and grow. You only chose the best strategies that can help you reach your target results. They contain all the positive ideas that you need to successfully carry out your proceedings. You have the choice of buttons, but what you must put in mind is that life is like the 2 sides of a coin.

This toolkit can be people, organizations, or another thing that is filled with ideas. The people that have passed through the same road of life as you are here. Take this opportunity to explore them to feed you with ideas about what you are doing and how it can affect your mind. Don't give room for your mind to be easily exhausted and focused on one particular thing, be it good or bad. Big minds attract different ideas of what you can to keep yourself busy leaving no room for unnecessary behaviors that are risky to your wee being.
Bad Daycare

How you spend your day has a great impact on your personal welfare. When you spend your entire day doing nothing or engaging in activities that do not add progress to your life, then you are surely wasting your life. Bad daycare includes spending your entire day doing one thing. Whatever it is that you are doing with your day, whether productive or nonproductive, will still affect your well if it is not properly managed.

Everyone have great minds and good ideas. The difference is how they channel their ideas and thoughts. Some people will share with others to get support or advanced ideas on how these things work in order for them to move forward. On the other hand, another person will choose to keep their ideas to them because they fear being criticized by the public. This will only stop them from making progress.

Let other people badmouth you for being real and true to yourself and everyone, rather than pleasing everyone to win their love. You will win their love yes, but will you be happy with what you have done by the end of the day, if no, then think twice before you make up your mind.

Comfort Zone

No one succeeds in life when they are stuck to their comfort zones. Learn to walk out of your comfort zone and try something new that makes you sweat. You will feel like you are hurting yourself, but the end result will convince you that you chose the best option and that you can prosper with it. That thing that everyone is afraid to try to face it boldly and give it a trial. You might just be opening another gate for your success.

They fear of trying something hard only keeps us revolving around one place but not making any progress. Many people always want to face things the easy way. They don't want to face the hard side of life. You may look at these people and think that they are living a good life and enjoying their comfort, but the truth is that these people are suffering the fear of struggling. This is the hardest battle you can ever fight in the journey of success.

Understand What Supports Me

We all need to understand the pillars of our wellbeing. What gives us the courage and strength to keep going and never look back is what contributes highly to our wellbeing. After we get in line with what supports us, we should take good care of it so that its impacts are not underrated, and its support is well maintained for our own satisfaction.

When we don't recognize what supports us, we risk losing its support when its presence is taken away from us. This support might be coming from the people who value us too much and want the best for us. For example, your parent can notice a talent in you that will contribute to your good lifestyle and offer to support you nurture this talent, but if you are showing zero interest in it, they can give up supporting you and focus on your other siblings who are ready to learn from them and appreciate their support.

Challenging Self-Care

Self-care is not an easy task as t sounds. You may not know how to go about everything to maintain a good life, free from drama and unnecessary stress. Some people struggle to live a better lifestyle than others without a single idea if what they are doing. They feel uncontended with their physical appearance and wish to do better than this, but they don't know how to go about it to the land where they want.

Life becomes difficult for them because they try everything possible to change from where they are to a better level, but unfortunately, they don't know how to do it because they don't even know what they are fighting. They do everything blindly, hoping that one day they will come to achieve what they want and live the comfortable life that they desire. The struggle of maintaining their well-being becomes a trial and error type of struggle.

Chapter 7: Reiki Symbols And Their Unique Uses

One of the fastest methods by which to connect a person with their higher energies is through the implementation of special signs, known as Reiki symbols.

Reiki symbols allow people to take their training to the next level, by allowing practitioners to use the energy of Reiki for a specific purpose.

In most instances, symbols really only affect the subconscious. But in Reiki, the symbols work very differently because they attune both the mind and body to Reiki energy in such a way as to allow the practitioner to activate the power of Reiki in its entirety. This is done by Reiki practitioners visualizing the symbols of Reiki, saying them aloud, or even drawing them. By using intention in the activation process, a Reiki practitioner can unlock the power of energy that the system encompasses.

To understand Reiki, it is important to know the meaning of each symbol. To start with, let's focus on the key symbols:
Cho Ku Rei: The Power Symbol

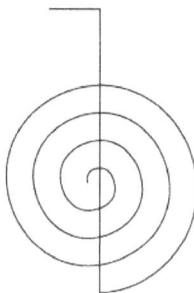

If you're looking for a fluctuation in power, whether that means an increase or decrease, Cho Ku Rei is the symbol for that corresponds to this.

The symbol represents chi, or the transfer of energy throughout the body.

When visualizing the power symbol, the Reiki practitioner instantly has a greater ability to illuminate, enlighten, and channel energy in their body.

How/When to Use Cho Ku Rei

The practice and use of Cho Ku Rei is most commonly found at the start of a Reiki session because the method is a potent way by which to boost Reiki power. The symbol can be implemented during a session too, in order to provide a quick boost of energy.

In addition, Cho Ku Rei can be used effectively to help the healing of an injury. Use of the symbol has been known to greatly assist with the healing of anything from light aches and pains to more serious and painful injuries.

And, in a more abstract sense, Cho Ku Rei can also be used while clearing negative energy. This can be taken a step further, as drawing the symbol on the walls of rooms can foster both light and positive energy within a household.

Cho Ku Rei can also be used effectively within your relationships with people too. It might be a good idea to have a picture of the Cho Ku Rei symbol on your business card, and working with it before a job interview will enhance your charisma. And, visualizing the symbol while having an important conversation with loved ones, is a great way to enhance compassion and connectivity.

The symbol has also been used as a protective talisman against misfortunes. Cho Ku Rei can purify negative energy, protecting the Reiki practitioner from adverse effects due to exposure of such energies.

This symbol is also known to be efficient in removing any traces of negative energy from the food that you are about to consume.

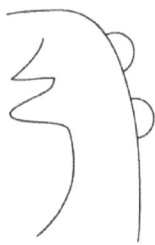

Sei He Ki: The Harmony Symbol

The power of the Sei He Ki symbol resides within its ability to bring emotional balance and promote mental clarity.

The word Sei He Ki means "God and man become one". The drawn symbol resembles either a wave cresting and preparing to crash. It can also be shown as a bird's wing.

The symbol is known for its ability to balance both sides of the brain, bringing about equilibrium.

In addition to being known as a stability/harmony symbol, Sei He Ki is also portrayed as a protection symbol.

How to Use Sei He Ki

If you want to improve your memory, Sei He Ki will be of great use to you. For example, you could draw this symbol on the pages of your notebook, or a book that you're reading, in order to retain the necessary information for as long as possible.

Another way of activating the Reiki symbol Sei He Ki is by using the technique of visualization. Simply imagine the symbol sitting atop your head as you focus your mind. This practice attunes your spiritual and vibrational alignment to the frequency of the symbol, enticing the symbol to activate and share its transformational power with you.

Additionally, if you're struggling to kick a bad habit like excessive drinking or smoking, overeating, etc. consider calling on Sei He Ki. Calling upon the symbol brings focus and increases your self-worth, putting you on target for success.

For those who suffer from headaches, Sei He Ki will help by balancing out the instability, which very often is the reason for them. It will relieve the headache and there will be no need to take unnecessary medicine.

Sei He Ki also provides protection from negative vibes, working as a protective symbol.

Another very important moment is that Sei He Ki can make your affirmations stronger and more powerful. If you're writing down your affirmations, my advice is to try drawing this symbol next to them — it will enhance them, and they will be more likely to bring the necessary results!

Hon Sha Ze Sho Nen: The Distance Symbol

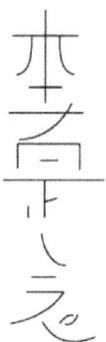

The symbol, Hon She Ze Sho New has one of the most complex meanings of all the symbols.

Hon She Ze Sho Nen is a transcendental symbol, which translates to "having no present, past, or future".

The symbol serves the main function of harnessing and sending Reiki energy across time and space — whether that be the past, present, or future.

A great example of how the symbol works can be found within its ability to heal old wounds without changing the past. While the past or events of the past cannot be changed in a physical sense, the effects of past experiences — which can live within our psyche — can be reframed using the symbol. This reframing allows the Reiki practitioner to take what was once pain that felt unjust, and turn it into a powerful and transformational learning lesson.

How to Use Hon Sha Ze Sho Nen

While the symbol is considered one of the most powerful, it has to be used with precision, in order to work. The symbol works more effectively on the mental and spiritual body, much more so than it does on the physical body. Reiki experts suggest using this symbol on a day-to-day basis, especially if you need to effectively encourage past and future healing on the body.

Dai Ko Myo: The Master Symbol

This symbol is one of the most nourishing and enlightening of all the Reiki symbols. It has the highest vibration, and heralds the most potent ability for transformation.

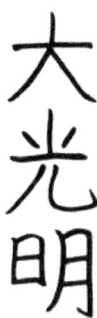

Dai Ko Myo has powers to heal and transform a Reiki practitioner in ways that are truly all-encompassing. The symbol can promote dynamic healing of the chakras (spiritual energy systems of the body), and the soul.

The symbol means "great enlightenment" or "bright shining light".

Use of this symbol is synonymouswith elevating the practitioner's state of being, helping them to rise up past their old self, bringing them into direct alignment with their positive/higher self, and ultimately bringing them closer to God/the Universe.

How to Use Dai Ko Myo

To call upon the maximum effects of Dai Ko Myo, these are some of the methods you could use.

The first is to draw the symbol. Another is to visualize the completed symbol. The last is to visualize or draw it with your third eye.

You can also meditate with the Dai Ko Myo symbol. This will nourish your body and soul, giving you the power to help not only yourself but others around you.

If you're working on improving your relationship with yourself and want to achieve more self-awareness or a stronger spiritual practice, this symbol is an important one to call upon. You can use it in combination with other Reiki symbols, it will only make it more effective.

Dai Ko Myo is also a great way to help strengthen your immune system. Since Dai Ko Myo improves the energy flow throughout the entire body, it can effectively help clear blockages. This in effect cleans, purifies, and enhances the efficiency of your immune system, which in turn increases your overall health exponentially.

Raku: The Completion Symbol

The Raku symbol, or the "Fire Serpent," as it is known by meaning, is a symbol used at a very advanced level in Reiki.

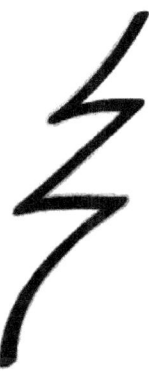

The symbol is drawn in a zigzag, lightning-bolt-like, shape. It is used to ground or center a practitioner after a Reiki session.

The purpose of Raku is to allow the body to receive the benefits of Reiki. It is similar to the way Shavasana is used at the end of a yoga session to help the body absorb all the benefits of the practice.

Raku is also a grounding symbol, and it is often used by Reiki practitioners to clear any negative energy they may have collected from the person they were practicing on or to rid themselves of any negative energy that they have cultivated within themselves.

How to Use Raku

You can use this symbol at the end of a Reiki practice, in order to ground yourself and absorb all the benefits of the energy transfer. Besides, when you find yourself in need of a moment of grounding in day-to-day life, feel free to draw the Raku, too.

How to Use Multiple Reiki Symbols at Once

Reiki symbols can be used individually or in conjunction with each other. By combining the power of multiple symbols, a truly powerful synergy can be formed.

A great example of this multiple usage can be found in the practice of healing a sick individual. The Reiki practitioner can start by holding a photograph of the person in question. Then they must focus their attention on the Cho Ku Rei, Sei Hei Ki, and Hon Sha Ze Sho Nen symbols, a total of three seconds per symbol, for three repetitions. Finally, the practitioner must recite the recipient's name 3 times while still holding their photograph. This method is a very powerful healing technique that demonstrates the potent mix of healing energy that the Reiki symbols can invoke.

Another great way to use several different symbols at once is by sending Reiki energy out toward a future event that you're apprehensive or nervous about. Anything from a job interview, doctor's appointment, impending results of a medical test or academic exam, the list goes on.

This is done by three repetitions of reciting the names Cho Ku Rei, Sei He Ki, Hon Sha Ze Sho Nen. As the practitioner does this, it is important that they close their eyes and visualize the shapes of each of the symbols. This will invoke vibrations of great calm and peace, something that will extend out into the rest of the day. This process brings control of your day to you. The positivity sparked by the process gives you power over what has passed and what will pass that day, letting you be an instigator of positivity, as opposed to a victim of circumstance. The process sharpens your senses too, as you become the conductor, and not just the audience, in the symphony of your life.

Chapter 8: Chakras And Reiki

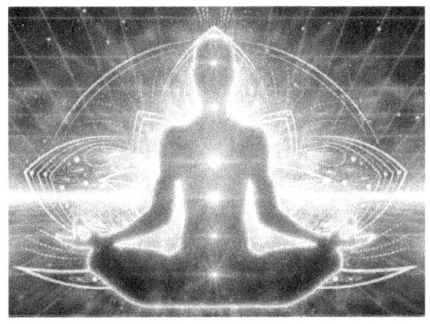

The chakra system is a huge component of the energetic anatomy in the body. It is the convergence point of the physical body, energetic body, and the emotional body. Chakras are pools of energy, or energetic centers that help the overall energetic flow within the three bodies that make up a person, that make up you.

Since the chakras are primary sources of energy, then they resonate well with Reiki energy. Since an imbalanced chakra can lead to dis-ease and many uncomfortable or debilitating symptoms in the body, and

Reiki energy is a healing method that balances energy in the body, then Reiki can help balance the chakras and some root sources of imbalance.

In the human body there are as many as one hundred and fourteen chakras that make up the chakra system. In western traditions and energetic healing, seven chakras known as the 'main chakras' are the focus of energetic healing.

Each of these chakras resonates with a body cavity, emotions, colors, organs, glands, and hormones. These associations are what lead to the manifestation of symptoms when a chakra is imbalanced. Knowing what the chakra associations are can better help you understand what chakras need work or focus.

Since Reiki is intuitive and goes where it is needed, you aren't going to direct the Reiki energy towards a chakra for balancing. However, knowing where the imbalance has occurred can help guide you to the cause of the imbalance. Once it is realigned with Reiki energy, you can work towards making shifts in your life that will prevent the imbalance from coming back.

Most Reiki courses do include information on the chakras. For more in-depth discussion on knowledge on the chakras and chakra healing, be sure to check out another book in this series Chakras Healing for Beginners. That book will elaborate on the information in this chapter and give you more knowledge and wisdom to help with balancing our chakras.

When you learn the different static hand positions for a Reiki session, you'll notice that they correspond to the chakras and the body cavities that the seven main chakras align with. This further illustrates how Reiki energy and the chakra system are related. Many Reiki practitioners might even start or end their sessions by placing their hands over the seven main chakras on themselves or on their recipient.

As touched on in a former chapter, the word chakra translates into wheel or disk. Chakras are spinning disks or wheels of energy in the body. They are cone shaped and expand outward, connecting the physical, emotional, and energetic bodies. The chakras have energy that rotates in a clockwise and counterclockwise direction creating a sort of three-dimensional spiral. Chakras are three-dimensional, hence their cone shape.

The seven main chakras run along the spin. The apex, or point of the cone is at the spine and then the chakra cones expand outwards to the front and back of the body. The exceptions to this are the crown chakra which only expands up out of the top of the head and the root chakra which expands down to the feet.

Crown Chakra

The crown chakra is located at the top of the head. It expands up from the cranium and into the universe. The crown chakra connects your personal energy to universal energies and cosmic energies. This is the source of your cosmic consciousness and connects you to divine intelligence and wisdom.

The crown chakra is associated with the color violet or white. It represents bliss, union, and the knowledge that you are one with all else. The crown chakra resonates with peace and cosmic consciousness.

The crown chakra is associated with the mind, brain, nervous system, and the pituitary gland. It is also associated with the hypothalamus. The crown chakra is an element-less chakra. Your crown chakra allows you to access higher states of consciousness and is connected to transcendence of your limitations. Opposites become one in the crown chakra. You can also receive clarity, enlightenment, and wisdom.

When the crown chakra is imbalanced it can present as many different symptoms. It creates feelings of disconnection for the spirit and spiritual energies. A cynical mood about what is sacred can be a result of an imbalanced crown chakra. You may also feel disconnected from your physical body. Other imbalances present as obsessive attachments to spirituality, being close minded, headaches, nightmares, mental illness, and eye problems.

When working with the crown chakra there are some crystals that can enhance the Reiki energy for balancing this chakra. Crystal associations include clear quartz, selenite, diamond, and amethyst.

Third Eye Chakra

Your third eye chakra is between your brows on the front of your body. On the back of your body, the third eye chakra is at the occipital ridge. Your third eye chakra is associated with intuition, awareness, and perception. It provides the energy for spiritual reflection and insights. Through the third eye chakra, you experience clear thought, visions, and independent thought in a strong mind.

The color associated with the third eye chakra is indigo or dark purple. It resonates with the cranial cavity of the body as well as the eyes, nose, and the ears. The third eye chakra resonates with the pituitary gland and helps to regulate hormone production. The third eye chakra is associated with all elements.

This is your intuitive center, your foresight. The third eye chakra is driven by imagination and open mindedness. It can help you see subtle qualities in reality and open you up to different realms and their energies. The third eye chakra closely resonates with dimensions and the spirit worlds. The third eye chakra is also associated with the development of psychic abilities and energetic shifts or movements.

When imbalanced, the third eye chakra can contribute to the feeling of being stuck in a rut. It prevents you from being able to look beyond your own problems. When overactive, the third eye chakra can cause a lack of support from the other chakras. It can create fantasies that are more real and desirable than reality. An imbalanced third eye chakra can also prevent you from being able to see visions of yourself. You might try to reject anything spiritual and have the inability to see the bigger picture. Imbalances can lead to a general lack of clarity, depression, anguish, and mental turmoil.

Crystals that can be used to enhance Reiki energy when working with the third eye chakra include amethyst, fluorite, kyanite, and lapis lazuli.

Throat Chakra

The heart chakra is located at the base of the throat on the front of the body. It is located at the base of the cervical vertebrae on the back of the body, or between two tops of the shoulder blades. Your throat chakra is your center of communication and expression. This is both verbal and non-verbal communication. It is your authentic voice, your truth.

The throat chakra is associated with the thoracic cavity. Its element association is spirit or ether. It resonates with the shoulders, neck, mouth, jaw, tongue, pharynx, larynx, vocal cords, palate, and thyroid gland. The thyroid gland regulates body temperature, growth, and metabolism. The color of the throat chakra is blue.

The throat chakra is all about expressing yourself and expressing your truth. It is closely related to the sacral chakra which is a center of creativity and expression of your identity. The throat chakra is a reference point that connects and aligns with all the body chakras, including main chakras and sub-chakras. In your throat chakra, external and internal communication take place. It also provides you with a connection to etheric realms and helps you to create, bring projects ideas and blueprints into a reality.

When imbalanced, the symptoms of the throat chakra can present as a lack of control with speech. This can be speaking too much or too little, or speech impediments. With an imbalanced throat chakra, you might have difficulty listening to other people or listening to the universe. You may have difficulty keeping secrets, or be very secretive. It can also manifest as compulsive or excessive lying and not being able to keep your word. Other imbalances in the throat chakra include stiff neck, hearing problems, sore throat, and thyroid problems.

Crystals that resonate with the throat chakra include blue lace agate, lapis lazuli, blue jade, blue topaz, and celestite. These crystals can enhance Reiki energy work with the throat chakra.

Heart Chakra

Your heart chakra is located in the center of your sternum in the front of your body and between the center of your shoulder blades, just above the adrenal glands, on the back of your body. It is not directly over the heart organ. The heart chakra is the center of unconditional love and compassion. This is love for yourself, for others, romantic love, familial love, friend love, and an all-encompassing universal love.

Associated with the color green, the heart chakra resonates with the element air. It is closely associated with the diaphragm between the thoracic and abdominal cavities. The heart chakra resonates with the thymus and the lymphatic system. It also correlates to the heart organ, diaphragm, and the lungs. The heart chakra is driven by integration and transformation. It is a bridge between earthly and spiritual aspirations.

Your heart chakra is going to give you deep feelings of connection. It provides harmonious exchanges of energy with everything and everyone around you. It also allows you to see the world and everything in it from a place of love and beauty. A healthy, balanced heart chakra opens you up to giving and receiving love. It is a pure source of unconditional, universal love for everyone and everything, detached from personal biases.

If the heart chakra becomes imbalanced it can lead to difficulty relating to other people and their emotions. Imbalanced heart chakras lead to excessive jealousy, codependency, and being closed down and withdrawn. Other imbalances in the heart chakra can lead to a lack of self-love, lack of self-worth, and a lack of self-confidence. This can lead to fear and self-destructive tendencies.

When working with Reiki and the heart chakra some crystals that can enhance the healing process include rose quartz, green jade, emerald, green calcite, malachite, and rhodonite.

Solar Plexus Chakra

The solar plexus chakra, sometimes called the naval chakra or the third chakra, is located an inch or two above the naval on the front of the body. On the back of the body, the solar plexus chakra is an inch or two above the sacrum in the center of the back. The solar plexus chakra is your will center, your personal power, and your assertiveness. It is the center of yourself, your identity.

From the solar plexus chakra, you get control. You get control over your own path, destiny, and dreams. The solar plexus chakra is associated with the color yellow. Its element is fire, and this is where the term 'fire in your belly' comes from. The solar plexus chakra resonates with the abdominal cavity and the organs that reside there. It is closely related to your stomach, intestines, and the digestive system. It is your center of personal power and will power.

Your inner child resides in your solar plexus chakra. It is also the source of power for your mental abilities and activates your ability to assert yourself into the world. The idea of 'making your mark' in the world comes from your solar plexus chakra. You have a purpose in the world and your solar plexus chakra can help lead you to it. The solar plexus is your personal identity. It is where your assuredness, self-discipline, and independence stems from.

When imbalanced, the solar plexus chakra can lead to symptoms that result in energetic, physical, mental, and emotional illnesses. This includes obsessive compulsive disorders and control issues. An imbalanced solar plexus chakra might present with poor decision-making skills, problems with the immune system and the nervous system as well as low virality.

If you are using Reiki to work with the Solar Plexus chakra, some crystals that can enhance the experience include yellow tourmaline, yellow topaz, pyrite, tiger's eye, and citrine.

Sacral Chakra

Your sacral chakra is located about an inch below your naval on the front of your body and right over your sacrum on the back of your body. The sacral chakra is your pleasure center. It is the source of your passions and desires. This chakra is also associated with sensuality and sexuality. It is sometimes called the sex chakra or the second chakra.

Orange is the color of the sacral chakra and water is its element. The sacral chakra is associated with the abdominopelvic cavity and organs such as the bladder, uterine tract, and other low abdomen organs. It's also associated with the adrenal glands and helps regulate and maintain the immune system. Descriptions for the sacral chakra include flowing and flexible. It is strongly connected to the emotional body which contributes to creativity, pleasure, and sensuality. It is driven by pleasure and the pleasure principle.

The sacral chakra is your emotional center. This is where your sexual orientation and expression of sexual desires stems from. Since it is motivated by pleasure, your sacral chakra is going to encourage you to enjoy life through all of your senses. It wants you to experience the world around you through taste, touch, sound, smell, sight. The sacral chakra is connected to the throat chakra as it is a source of expressing your personal identity. It also supports personal expansion and growth as well as creativity and fantasies.

If the sacral chakra becomes imbalanced, it can present as dependency or codependency on people or substances. You might find yourself being ruled by your emotions or be completely numb and out of touch. Imbalances in the sacral chakra can lead to overindulgences in fantasies. There can be a manifestation of obsessions with sexual intimacy or a lack of interest in sex. You might feel stuck in one mood. Other imbalances in the sacral chakra present as boredom, over-seriousness, resentment, disdain, as well as bladder and uterine disorders.

Crystals that resonate with the sacral chakra and can enhance your Reiki sessions include copper, jasper, carnelian, amber, moonstone, and orange calcite.

Root Chakra

The root chakra is located at the base of the spine. It extends downwards toward the feet. This is your grounding center, your foundation. The root chakra is sometimes called the first chakra. It is linked to your security and survival.

The element of the root chakra is earth and it is a dense chakra. The root chakra is associated with the color red and sometimes black. It resonates with the pelvic cavity and the organs within. The root chakra resonates with the reproductive organs of both men and women, as well as the reproductive hormones. It regulates production as well as sexual development.

Your root chakra is the source of your security. It is the foundation of yourself and for the expansion and growth of life. It is your support system for growth and your anchor for your energies to this world. The root chakra holds your basic needs for survival and is a major contributor to your physicality. It grounds you and holds many aspects of yourself, at least the aspects that make up your foundation.

When imbalanced, the root chakra contributes to excessive negativity. You might become cynical and live inside your illusions. This is often accompanied by feelings of dread and insecurity. You can get trapped in a survival mindset, fight or flight mode. You may become fearful and paranoid. Other symptoms of an imbalanced root chakra include eating disorders, obesity, hemorrhoids, constipation, and any issues with the blood, bones, feet, and legs.

If you are using Reiki energy to work with the root chakra, some crystals that resonate with the root chakra include smoky quartz, garnet, ruby, black tourmaline, obsidian, jet, and onyx.

Chapter 9: Balancing The Chakra Forces

The recovery of the balanced energy flow of the chakras is known as, "chakra balancing." This is a feeling of increased energy, relaxation, wellness, and healthiness.

In this process of balancing, certain chakras on the body that are known to be particularly powerful points of energy are returned to a balanced state. Each individual chakra is part of a system that works together as a group. They connect with each other, and when they are all in harmony, they end up overflowing with energy.

When working with this system, it is important to connect with each energy chakra, as well as the areas that surround them. The key to a healthy mind and body is opening and balancing the chakras to create a sustainable energy flow, to restore your overall health and well-being.

The chakras are centered on the physical body and can be awakened through a meditation process, or the energy transfer process from another person to yourself. The most common ways to balance your chakras are:

- Meditation (including chakra meditation)
- Exercises focused on connecting the mind and body, i.e., yoga
- Breathing exercises, i.e., pranayama (Hindu yoga)
- Holistically via alternative medicine
- Hands-on via energy healing

Common practices to restore chakra system balance are:

- Reiki healing
- Craniosacral therapy (gentle touch therapy to the cranium joints)
- Pranic healing (energy healing)
- Use of chakra healing stones

The purpose of balancing is to achieve a uniform flow that will continue to provide an overall level of energy. Every day, we are faced with many causes of stress, and demands resulting in energy level changes. Some changes are completely draining, and some are filled with nourishing energy. By managing our energy each day, we can create a more steady overall balance of energy that will then help to contribute to our overall feeling of wellness.

Chakra imbalances caused by demands and stress will create interruptions in our flow of energy. A chakra imbalance can affect:

- The amount of energy flowing through the chakra system, that can cause either balance or imbalance.
- Energy flow, if not maintained at a constant level by the chakras, will become overactive, or imbalanced.
- The energy field will become imbalanced if the chakra positions are moved out of their proper alignment. Balancing establishes sufficient and consistent flow of the body's energy, and is crucial to long-term health. It will naturally try to regulate and realign where there's distortion or displacement.

As our souls learn and live life in numbered incarnations, we usually learn and unevenly grow which create an imbalance in the soul. Healing occurs when we resolve inner conflicts that create spiritual, mental, and emotional pain. These imbalances and balances in our souls are mirrored in:

- Our feelings and thoughts
- Our emotional well-being and our mental and physical health
- Our chakras' colors, sizes, and shapes
- Things that are challenging for us and things that we find easy
- Things in our life that we have too much of or things we lack
- The many different people in our lives
- The way we feel about the universe
- The world all around us

Our souls will grow in life, and we can seek a higher understanding, health, happiness, balance, and peace along a learning path. All of us are divine souls even if we don't acknowledge our spiritual essence.

By making a promise of understanding, we can help ourselves get rid of our pain and fears so they can truly rise to the surface and be healed once and for all. Some mental attitudes can be changed simply by understanding a known truth concerning ourselves. Other problems might be ingrained so deeply that is hard to be objective about how we really feel about them. Also, a lot of searching of the soul, meditation, determination, reflection, and prayer may be required to invoke positive change, to achieve a resolution of problems. These issues are inevitably released and then are healed slowly but surely.

We are all divinely guided when we are on a journey to heal, but sometimes it takes courage to persevere and get to the heart of the matter in order to face these difficult issues once and for all. Sometimes we think we have dealt with and released these issues, thinking that they are gone for good. However, unexpectedly, they appear right in front of us again. Once we know in our spiritual mind that they are gone; they are gone for good. This is sometimes not a fast solution, but it is the real way to a permanent one.

Power is the highest part of the consciousness of the universe. It is thought also to be a supreme state of enlightenment. After many lifetimes, our bodies learn that inner balance creates happiness and harmony, and imbalance brings suffering and pain. We usually grow unevenly which brings pain and imbalance that tells our consciousness to grow in those areas that have been ignored for years due to fear or laziness. People, events, and situations throughout our life create fears that are deeply ingrained within us, but they present us with opportunities to face them, overcome them, learn and grow from them.

Although in most lifetimes there will be suffering and pain, we can work to overcome them and understand that we are blessed with unlimited amounts of potential for happiness and love. Finding out about ourselves, our relationships with others, and that the universe brings love and wisdom, will all help us get to where we need to be.

Reiki treats the entire body, including the mind, spirit, and emotions. When given a treatment by a Reiki practitioner, the body and mind relax, and the energy begins to flow throughout the body, resulting in a feeling of being lighter and uplifted. It focuses on relaxing the patient and getting in tune with their innermost self. It focuses on letting the world go and bringing in the light of peace and health.

Chapter 10: Forgiveness Letter

Forgiving someone or oneself is an opportunity to let go of anger and pain built inside you. Built up emotions only brings unhappiness and depression. Forgiving is not forgetting. You cannot forget the incident or people that hurt you. But forgiving lets you free yourself from built up emotions of anger and hurt. Forgiving is burying all the grudges and move on with your life.

Same way, if you have hurt someone, now is the time to apologize. Sometimes it so happens that writing brings out better emotions than being verbal. So go and ask for forgiveness now and forgive to move on with your life. If for some reason you can't say sorry or give forgiveness directly, here is the reiki method. Forgiveness letter. Write different letter for different person.

1.Be alone. Switch off your phone. Lit a candle in front of you.

2.Take pen and paper. Draw CKR on 4 corners. Think of the person you want to forgive or ask forgiveness.

3.Write your letter. Describe the incident, your feelings about it, how it will make you feel after forgiving or apologizing. Pour your heart into the letter.

4.Take a light colored crayon or color pencil and draw CKR, chanting its name thrice. Imagine gliding CKR in that person's heart. Same way draw SHK and HSZSN over the letter with crayon or light colored pencil, chant its name thrice and glide symbols in his/her heart.

5.Draw another HSZSN in front of you. Connect HSZSN to the person.

6.Read out loud your letter. Burn the letter. Imagine all the resentment and anger burning along with the letter. If it's granting forgiveness letter, say I FORGIVE _____ thrice. If it's an apology letter say I AM SORRY. PLEASE FORGIVE ME _____ thrice.

7.Stay alone for a while. Pay attention to your thoughts. Feel the peace within you. You will surely feel light- hearted.

Following the same ritual, you can release your karma. For karma release, write "Dear creator, father, mother, son as one... If any of my ancestors, relatives or myself has offended you, your relatives or ancestors across any life time, we ask for your forgiveness".

Miraculous Reiki Chi Ball- Case Story

Chi Ball is my personal favorite method for healing and manifesting goals. Most of you must be aware of what Chi Ball is. A Reiki Chi Ball is one of the method for distant healing in which you make an energy ball and release it to Universe.

Before starting this amazing and miraculous case story, I want to thank Ananya Sen for introducing and teaching this amazing method to me.

Thank You Ananya.

I was with my friend and kids at home, just having fun and good time. I got a call from a client, totally distressed. Her daughter Honey missed her exam. She was preparing her submission work for college and hence slept late. When she woke up in the morning, she had unbearable headache. She thought of taking a nap but unfortunately she could not wake up on time. Honey went to her Sir and requested him to re-schedule her exam.

The Sir refused bluntly. That's when my client Vinny called me. She asked me to 'do something'- "Do whatever you can but please do something".

I made a Reiki Chi Ball. Invoking symbols, Archangels and Honey's guides. While creating this energy ball, I kept a constant flow of symbols. I imagined all 4 symbols flowing constantly to Reiki Chi Ball, floating in the Chi ball. I released the Reiki Chi Ball with the simple intention that 'Honey wrote her exam today'. Nothing more, nothing less.

Within 15-20 minutes, I got a call from Vinny (client) that Honey is allowed to write her exams. According to Honey, She was sitting distraught and suddenly her Sir came and gave permission to re-plan her exam the next day. She was amazed and awe-struck with this sudden change of situation. I sent one more Reiki Chi Ball with lots symbols, to the sir (I don't know the name) with the intention to soften his heart. So, again within half an hour I got a call from Vinny, saying Honey is writing her exam today, NOW. The magic of miraculous Chi Ball working super-fast.

Meanwhile here at home, my friend and kids were all going gaga about the whole scenario and amazing Reiki Chi Ball. Reiki Chi Ball always helps me. Never failed so far. It is one of the most under-rated healing modality according to me. Thank You Miraculous Reiki Chi Ball for always helping me.

Psychic Surgery on Pet- Case Story

When Psychic surgery is merged with Reiki, it brings miraculous healing. Psychic surgery is non-invasive non-surgical surgery performed to remove negativity, blockage, and drainage from energy field and body. It is safe and non-painful method. Psychic surgery can be done on animals and plants too. Here on Reiki Rays we have infographic of Psychic Surgery technique.

I have performed Psychic Surgery many times on various people. Few days back, I performed first time on my pet. My dog PARI was unwell. I could not make out what was wrong with her. She was feeling down, not at all playful and she did not eat for the whole day. On the first day I thought it is her usual eating tantrum. On second day I got worried as she didn't even touch her breakfast and lunch. I gave her reiki with the intention that the energy flows wherever it is needed the most. Still she did not touch her dinner. On the third day I called up her vet and he told me to wait and watch. But still, being a 'mommy' I was worried. I tried giving treats to her that she never refuse. She did not even touch her treat. I again gave her reiki with the same intention. I was quite confused as why no change in her even after receiving healing. Generally she accepts healing very openly, never runaway and it always used to work.

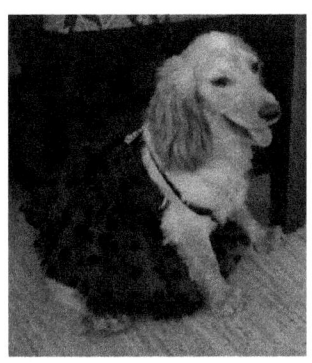

I could not see her feeling so down and not at all playful. On day four, I scanned her aura with the helpof Byosen scanning method while she was sleeping. I found disturbance around her solar-plexus chakra and sacral chakra. I had been giving her reiki since 2 days and found no change in her so I started wondering how to heal her. I prayed to my angels and guides asking them how to heal my Pari. I got reply in an instant. Just one word reply. Psychic Surgery. Without giving a second thought, I performed psychic surgery on Pari. I removed all the blockages and accumulated debris from her body and energy field. Then I protected her with DKM. Within five minutes of psychic surgery, she woke up and vomitted. I and my daughter(leve 2 reiki) both understood that this is just negativity and blockages coming out. In no time she was her playful self again and to my sheer relief she finished her food too.

Reiki helps me in numerous ways in my regular routine day to day life. Thank You Reiki☐

Quick Aura Cleansing Techniques

Our Aura is like a magnet. It attracts all kinds of energies surrounding us. We cannot always be surrounded by good people and positive environment. It isn't always possible to avoid things that leaves negative vibes in or aura. Due to work, travel, or for whatever reason you come across and pass negative vibes too. All these negative vibes get accumulated to our aura. So it is very essential to cleanse our aura on regular basis. There are many techniques to cleanse aura like Kenyo Ku, Sweeping, and Smudging etc. Below are some simple and easy techniques to cleanse aura.

☐If you have a bath tub, fill the bath tub with warm water. Add some essential oil.

Add Himalayan salt or sea salt. Invoke reiki symbols and start reiki flow. Intend that this water will clear all negativity away, cleanse your aura and fill it with light. Light small candle and burn incense stick. Step in your bath tub and relax.

☐ It is a variation of the above method if you do not have bath tub. In a bucket, add essential oil and Himalayan Salt or Sea Salt. Invoke reiki symbols and start reiki flow with the intention to remove negativity and remove aura. Have a bath with this water.

☐ Draw reiki symbols on shower head and give reiki to shower head with the intention that the water that flows out will remove all negativity and remove aura. Imagine water coming out of shower head a sparkling white light and covering you in divine light.

☐ Draw Cho Ku Rei on the roof of your mouth with your tongue and hold your tongue there. Breathe in deeply through your nose while counting till 6. Count till 3. Exhale through mouth counting till 6 with lips slightly pressed together. Do this 3 times. This is a real quickie to cleanse your aura.

☐ Draw reiki symbols on a smudge stick, hold it in your palms and give reiki for few seconds with the intention that the smoke that comes out will remove all negative, dirt and debris from your aura.

Burn the end of the smudge stick and wait till the flame is out. Now, waft all around your body from head to toe. The smoke will cleanse your aura.

☐ Draw reiki symbols on palms and set your intention to cleanse aura. Now with your fingers, comb through your aura from head to toe, untangling wherever you feel any tangles or heaviness in energy.

☐ Soak any flower (rose, jasmine, lavender) in distilled water for couple of hours. Fill the water in spray bottle. Charge it with reiki and sprinkle on your client from head to toe. Move clockwise and spray water at your client's front, back and both sides- top to bottom. They will feel extremely refreshed.

☐ Take a raw unbroken egg and wash it. Infuse with reiki. Say any prayer and set your intention. Sweep your aura with this egg starting from head to toe. Some prefer egg contact on skin and some prefer noncontact method. You can hold the egg for longer on certain spots if you detect dark energies. Once finished, break the egg n flush. Some prefer doing egg-reading. They can break the egg in water bowl and let it set for few hours. DO NOT COSUME THIS EGG.

☐Imagine white or golden light covering your aura, passing through your crown and out through feet, taking away all negativity and blockages.

☐Imagine violet flame in front of you. Step into the flame and let it cleanse your aura by removing negativity. When you feel it is done, protect yourself with CKR.

☐Give a chi-ball to self with the intention to keep your aura clean and chakras unblocked.

In all of the above techniques you must have noticed that having a strong intention is the main thing. Cleansing your aura is MUST. Cleanse your aura regularly to stay healthy and happy☐

Chapter 11: Reiki And Related Concepts

Karuna Reiki

The question of 'suffering' is central to the discourse of many enlightening religions, as it radically defines what it means to be human in a world of pleasure and pain, highs and lows, and a constant search for finding meaning in the labyrinthine cycles of existence. The word Karuna has its roots in the Sanskrit language and holds immense importance in Hinduism and Buddhism. A translation of it would mean "compassionate action." This compassion is amalgamated with good deeds to achieve completion as human beings in this world, and dissipate the universal suffering faced by all species. The idea of equality is central to such belief systems, and therefore, all those who achieve enlightenment view each person as being a valuable part of a whole without any distinctions in treatment.

The act of extending Karuna to every individual is viewed as a naturalistic assumption in these schools of thought. It is based on the belief that the act of kindness that one shows while helping others is the ultimate virtue in this world because it heals the wounds of those who need a remedy. The idea of love is, of course, a guiding factor, yet even when one employs rationality; it is quite lucid that it is the best course of action to take if one wants to live in tranquility. The system of Karma, which is central to the belief system of Hinduism postulates that an individual's life is a reflection of their past deeds and actions. Therefore, it is only prudent to give to others, what one must expect to receive from them. Which is to say, if humans want to be loved, they must give love in return. 'Parjana,' which is translated as "wisdom" is enshrined in Buddhist religious literature, and postulates that Karuna must be amalgamated with wisdom to produce emancipation from the alienating conditions produced by humanity.

Individuals who have successfully achieved enlightenment must base the ideology of their lives on the idea of Karuna, and look at it as the source of their motivation for the annihilation of all suffering in this world. It is an enduring quality that must be cultivated by all those who aim to receive healing, and channel the energy it derives its strength from. Not only are teachers supposed to possess Karuna, but also students who aim to recover from the trauma of their existence. This hastens the process of emancipation and healing. The practice of "Karuna Reiki" clears a path for individuals to form intimate working connections with enlightened teachers and leaders, which consist of those present in a tangible physical form, as well as those in spirit.

The Practice of Karuna Reiki

The performance of Karuna Reiki can only be taken up by advanced practitioners in the method. It employs the use of symbols, which are taught to students so they can use them for healing. It is distinct from Usui Reiki and is considered more effective in terms of the amount of energy that is received by the students.

There are distinct kinds of symbols within the practice of Karuna Reiki, which is divided into two distinct halves, namely, Karuna One and Karuna Two. Both of them consist of an equal number of symbols, and in totality, there are eight of them, which are employed in the healing process.

Karuna One Symbols

Zonar

This symbol aims at deconstructing problems that arise from a karmic or cosmic hitch in existence that could extend beyond our current dimension of existence. Since the idea of rebirth is central to religions such as Hinduism upon which Karmic theory is based, this symbol works towards healing the reminiscence of suffering from the past which has been carried to the present life. The Zonar symbol provides solace to those who suffer from karmic anguish and reorients the cells that cause pain.

Harth

Employed in the cure of cardiac issues, as well as the metaphysical sentimentality attached to the "heart," Harth is used in the reconciliation of relationships. All suffering accruing out of relationships of love, which include human connections as well as passions such as work, are healed through the Harth. It reinvigorates the whole aspects of desires and helps to deal with issues accruing out of addiction.

Halu

It is an advanced form of Zonar and has many far-reaching abilities of healing. It taps into multiple and deep dimensions of human existence. Since balance is central to the idea of healing, it restores exactly that and therefore reduces pessimistic patterns of behavior embedded in the subconscious. It adds immense lucidity to the lens individuals employ to uncover the truth of this world.

Rama

This symbol is used for orienting the chakras and balancing them by finding grounding for their functioning. It connects them to the deeper levels of the earth in a manner wherein negative energy is diluted. It creates a balance between the upper and lower chakras and orients them to function in tandem.

Karuna Two Symbols

Gnosa

It opens a pathway that helps the individual connect to their higher self. It exists to shun denial and increase self-awareness, which helps to expand the consciousness beyond the physicality of the human frame.

Kriya

The human species is afflicted with many trials and tribulations. The Kriya possesses holistic healing abilities and produces beneficial results when used with any of the seven chakras.

Lava

Since human realities are barely undiluted by external influences, there is often immense disillusionment faced by individuals. The Iava clears the human being's reality from such influence and helps it exist in its original undiluted form. It can also be employed for the healing of the earth.

Shanti

This symbol sieves the human being of all internalized ideas of negativity. It acts as a repellent of nightmares, traumas, fears, and produces tranquility in otherwise disturbed minds. It releases human beings from being shackled to the tiring complexities of their past and move forward as more peaceful individuals.

Karuna Reiki amalgamates the usage of these symbols to create the effect of healing on individuals through compassion and selflessness.

Kundalini Awakening

Kundalini is a form of repressed and dormant energy that is part of our body and flows through it. The premise of Kundalini energy is based on Hindu mythology, according to which Kundalini is a goddess in the form of a serpent who is present at the base of our spine, sleeping and lying dormant. Kundalini controls the first chakra, and lies coiled around it three times, literally holding it within her grasp. Kundalini holds within her the divine Kundalini Shakti – a literal representation of the energy that life itself holds, and it's her presence that gives life to all beings. Sometimes, Kundalini awakens and so does the energy she carries, slowly moving through the body as an upward snake-like force leading to the opening of all the chakras in the body.

This awakening of Kundalini is essential for it releases all the energy that was blocked in the first chakra and then goes on to pass this free energy through all the chakras, unblocking them and getting rid of all the negative energy that was situated in these chakras. This movement is intense, and people who experience this have to go through a lot of pain, but it's a heightened spiritual experience that leads to an opening of the mind. Kundalini awakening does not happen randomly but has to be stimulated through prolonged sacrifice in the form of yoga, meditation, fasting, and through psychedelic drugs. To understand it more simply, think of Kundalini as the force that water possesses when it falls from a great height – a sort of primal force that can eviscerate anything in its path. The release of this force leads to the creation of a network that connects all the chakras through the use of connections that already exist in our body, known as nadi, specifically, the central nadi known as Sushumna.

Although the purpose of Kundalini is to be a healing force, it can lead to unpleasant consequences and pain that can last up to a few months. Don't worry; if you are dealing with such effects, you can use the following tips to ease the unpleasantness:

Purify the Body

You have to rid your body of any impurities, such as recreational drugs, alcohol, caffeine, tobacco, or prescription drugs (unless they are necessary for survival). The food that you eat also adds to the impurity of your body, so avoid food with a lot of sugar and salt in it, processed food, greasy food, and preserved food. Eat wholesome food that rejuvenates the soul, and is high in protein content. Also, try to heal the body by getting a relaxing massage or by exercising.

Reduce Stress

Since Kundalini awakening is a huge spiritual change in your life, your mind and body don't have much energy to deal with things that are happening outside, since the inside is so stressful. So, make sure that you are stress-free during this period by ensuring necessary changes in your social environment.

Find Support

Support and solidarity are essential to face anything that happens in life. So, talk to people who are going through the same experience and knowledge of it, this way you can learn from their authority.

Educate Yourself

Knowledge can be empowering, especially when you're about to experience something you have never even heard of.

Read about Kundalini Awakening, nadis and Chakras.

Treat underlying psychological issues

Kundalini allows you to rework your whole body since there is a lot of change in energy; this is the best time to deal with any underlying psychological issues you may have. Face them with courage and resolve, and use the energy of the process to heal yourself.

Reiki and Kundalini Awakening

Kundalini Reiki is a specific form of Reiki that is concerned with the internal energy released by Kundalini. Through Reiki, you can harness this power, and awaken it slowly, gently, and most importantly, safely. If you are successful in this endeavor, Kundalini will rise and clear out all of your chakras, body layers, and energy networks. Reiki also helps to make this whole process smoother and faster by adding additional Reiki energy into the mix. The end goal of this exercise is to stretch the limits of consciousness by cleaning out the different layers of the body, which allows for a vibrant and deeper flow of energy.

Kundalini awakening is essential for growth and spiritual and personal development. Kundalini energy is situated in our First or Root Chakras, which is our sole connection to the energy of the Earth. This energy starts from the Root Chakras, passes through the major channels of energy, and goes out of the body through the Crown Chakra. Both of these Chakras control the whole flow of energy in the body, and they are linked together by the Sushumna, which disseminates energy to the rest of the chakras through its various tributaries known as 'stems.' Kundalini energy empowers the Sushumna, allowing it to stimulate power to all of the other chakras rejuvenating and enlivening the body. This energy also connects to our emotions and thoughts; so all this rush of positive energy clears the mind and emotions of all negativity.

Chapter 12: Twenty-Four Hand Positions In Reiki

After being attuned to Reiki First Degree, you become a Reiki Channel. What is attunement? Attunement, also known as initiation is the procedure through which the Reiki Master helps the student to become a Reiki Channel. One cannot get attuned to the Universal Energy on their own without the skilled supervision and guidance of the Master or the Mentor. On cannot become a Reiki Channel by simply learning from books. Just as you need to tune your radio to a certain wave length in order to access to your favorite program, your energy needs to be tuned in to the Universal Energy in order for you to benefit from its flow. Therefore, Reiki attunement is done with the help of your Reiki practitioner and strictly under his supervision.

The practice of Reiki helps us feed our energetic body. If our Life-energy is strong our physical body will naturally be strong and healthy. During a Reiki attunement the Reiki Teacher becomes the feeding bottle to the student's energy fields. The Reiki Teacher uses a definite formula to draw down Energy from the Universe

and then with the help of the sacred Reiki symbols, he activates the student's Chakras starting with the Crown Chakra.

The Reiki Teacher propels more energy into the Crown Chakra and slowly guides the Reiki Energy towards the Heart Chakra.

From there the Reiki Energy is slowly conducted towards the arms and hands and, through them, into the palms of the hands.

This newly created schema makes the student become a channel to the Universal Energy for life. Once attuned, Reiki Channels can immediately start drawing Reiki Energy without assistance and using it for their own benefit.

IMPORTANT STEPS FOR PRACTICING REIKI ON YOUR OWN

All the Reiki we will ever have will be in our hands. But then our hands are so small and our body so large! Therefore, in order to heal the whole body with your hands through the Reiki Healing System, Dr Usui established the treatment through the 24 hand positions. Before proceeding to practice Reiki, always bear in mind that you need to be completely relaxed with a peaceful disposition. There should be no disturbance either physical or mental. You can lie down or sit up, whichever feels comfortable to your. Start by a few deep breathing steps. Inhale through the nose, visualizing pure white light passing up into your nostrils and exhale slowly through your mouth, visualizing all your negative energy, in the form of a smoky cloud, leaving your body bit by bit.

Once you feel completely relaxed, rub your hands to activate energy. You will feel them becoming warm and balmy. You are now ready to start healing yourself. Invoke the Reiki Energy and start with the First Hand Position by laying your hands on your eyes. There are 24 positions in all consisting of all the major Chakras and some important parts of your body.

The 24 hand-positions should be practiced in the following order:

1. Eyes
2. Ears
3. Jaws
4. Temples
5. Back of the head
6. Back of the head and the forehead
7. Back of the neck and throat
8. Thymus and heart
9. Solar Plexus (stomach) and belly
10. Sacral Chakra (below the navel) and genitals.

Next we heal some organs, starting with:

11. Lungs
12. Liver and spleen
13. Intestines.

We move on to:

14. Joints of the legs.
15. Thighs
16. Knees
17. Calves
18. Ankles.
19. Soles of the feet.

We heal some back parts of the body:
20. Shoulders.
21. Upper back
22. Kidneys (waist)
23. Lower back.
24. Root Chakra

N.B: During the last Reiki hand-position, we heal the Root Chakra by placing both hands, one on top of the other, exactly on the areas between the anus and the genitals, thus giving this most important Chakra a double hand Reiki.

Reiki channels should bear in mind that while doing the 24 hand-positions, each position will need at least 3 minutes of hand application. You must heal every part of your body as listed above at least for 3 minutes. More would be better, but at least 3 minutes. This means that your whole body-healing treatment will last for about one to one and a half hours. You will have to practice Reiki Healing in this way for the next 20 days in order to complete twenty-one days of what we call the Cleansing Process.

The 21 Days Cleansing Process

In order to get full benefit from the practice of Reiki, it is compulsory to complete 21 days of Reiki practice for at least one and a half hour each day. You don't need to do it at the same time every day. Any time suitable to you will do. I often meet Reiki Channels who complain that they do not have enough time to devote to Reiki because of too hectic a schedule. To them I say that if they don't find time during the day they can spare an hour from their sleeping time. Yes, you can practice your Reiki just before going to sleep. After all it is your health which is the most important part of your life. Without it, nothing matters. Does it?

The 21 days of Reiki practice is a NECESSARY process because during this period Reiki will start to harmonize and balance your energetic system. This is also a crucial period where you start getting more and more flow of positive energy which progressively expels deeply-anchored negative energies accumulated in your core over time. These can be disease, stress, emotional imbalance or mental problems. As Positive Energy starts replacing the negative energy, you will feel you are going through a transformation—a change within your inner self. However, change does not come about without some sort of agitation and perturbation. Many people get disheartened, becoming almost unenthusiastic with the 21 days of cleansing process practice because they feel their existing problems (whether physical or mental) are increasing (sometimes dramatically) instead of abating and calming down. During the first few days of the 21 days of Reiki practice, some people may start having more discomfort or even become sicker. This should not mean that you should stop practicing your Reiki thinking that Reiki is the cause of their problem. In fact it is the other way round. It is very important for all Reiki Practitioners to explain to the students and patients they initiate that this early phase of discomfort is a part of the cleansing process and is only temporary. When negative energies start leaving your system, they do not do so quietly. In fact they cause considerable negative reactions while getting eliminated from your system. Some newly-started Reiki practitioners do get affected physically, emotionally or mentally. Problems which existed before taking attunement to Reiki look like they are erupting and flaring up. But this condition is temporary. If you fall sick during the early days of your 21 days practice, you can seek medical help to ease your problems; you can also take your medicines, but the practice should not be interrupted if you desire your negative energies to leave you for good. You will have to persevere. Your 21 days of Reiki practice should be completed at all cost. At the end of it, you will marvel at how well you will start feeling. You will get better and better in the course of the 21 days.

There are still a handful of cases where people in very poor health still don't feel better after completing their 21 days practice. Such people are advised to extend their practice for as long as it takes them until they completely achieve the harmony and balance needed to restore their health back. These cases can also be attended by their Reiki Teachers through their healing sessions or healing attunements to activate the process further.

After the 21 days cleansing process, you can still continue with the 24 hand positions everyday if you wish. Or else, you can do it twice or thrice a week until you feel ready to go for your Second Degree of Reiki. But remember that there is actually no need to hurry. People who rush through their Reiki Degrees, especially those who have long-term medical conditions, will not be doing themselves any good. This will look like the case where your doctor prescribed you 10 pills to be taken one per day but you go home gulp down the whole pack at once thinking that it will restore your health at once. This was just and an example of what may follow if your rush things during a healing process which in itself should be slow and soft.

Nothing off beam will happen if you rush through your Reiki Degrees; but in this process you might eventually miss the expected results and feel you have wasted both your time and money. No disease gets healed in a day. Reiki healing of the mind and the body needs time and patience. Reiki is no miracle pill. It is Divine Energy at work. Be patient, be attentive and follow your teacher's advice

Chapter 13: Optimizing The Benefits Of Reiki Healing

Let's talk specifics and how Reiki actually affects our body. Yes, it heals and hastens recovery. It calms our nerves and eliminates anxiety, but how does it do that? This is something that you need to understand in order to better perform it as well as further optimize the benefits it provides you with.

What Reiki does is raise your vibrational frequency which basically clears the blockages in your body that disrupts the proper flow of energy. This allows for healing to begin at the most basic component of your body, the cells.

As your healing progresses, this may lead to self-reflection, and you might find yourself assessing what led you to this point. If you have bad habits or certain addictions, Reiki might be able to help you overcome these, thus, allowing you to focus your energy to something more productive. This change, in turn, would only bring about more benefits and eventually, restore you to full health.

Of course, this can only happen if you allow it. The most important tenet associated with Reiki is a dedication to preserving one's own health. In this sense, the practitioners should embrace the simple fact that they themselves are responsible for their own well-being. Reiki only aids in that process.

The point is Reiki will not make you immune to the countless issues that you may face in life. It will not exempt you from the Natural Law so it is important that you take care of yourself properly. For example, should you injure yourself and don't take care of the wound, you will be inviting infection and other problems. Reiki healing will not magically get rid of that. You can try performing Reiki either before or after applying first-aid treatment to a wound or injury to help manage the pain and expedite the healing. Other medical interventions can further be applied depending on the situation. For example stitching might be required as well as antibiotics and/or supplements.

If you have an addiction like we previously mentioned, and don't make any effort towards changing and getting it out of your life, sooner or later you will suffer from the consequences. Even if you practice Reiki on yourself daily, you can't rely on it solely while you continue on living unhealthily. That is simply illogical.

The bottom line is simple: this practice is not an insurance policy. Instead it will aid you when it comes to taking care of your overall well-being by promoting change from the inside to the outside. And we all know that what is inside is more powerful and lasting than the transformations we do on the outside. With this in mind believe in the positive healing energy of Reiki and share it to all those you care.

Chapter 14: Tips

I want to go over a few tips with you than will help you in yourself Reiki sessions as well as sessions with clients.

The first tip I want to give you is that you should never rush a session. Most of the time you want to schedule a 60 minute session but allow yourself up to 90 minutes. Often you will find that Reiki practitioners try to rush through sessions in order to see more clients or they only focus on one specific symptom trying to treat it. This is not how Reiki works, make sure you take the time needed with each client. Some may not need a long period of time other will need longer sessions. Don't be greedy with Reiki.

Make sure when you are working with clients that you practice good hygiene. You are going to be in close contact with many different people and you want to make sure that your personal hygiene is up to par. You also want to make sure that you are washing your hands and your table after seeing each client. You don't want people spreading germs and clients getting sick every time they visit you.

Before you start a session with a client if you are going to be physically placing your hands on them you need to ask permission to do so. You also need to do whatever you can to keep your clients comfortable. You will be going over their entire body and this includes what some would call private areas on their body. Before you place your hands on these areas you need to ask your clients permission. An alternative is to hover your hands above the area but make sure the client knows what you are doing.

Often a client will become uncomfortable having someone's hands close to these areas. Another thing you can do is have the client place their hands over the area and hover your hand above theirs if it makes them feel more comfortable. Reiki is able to travel through their hands and able to travel the short distance from your hands hovering over their hands as well so they will not lose any benefit.

Do not skip these areas of the body just because it may make you are the client feel uncomfortable. The entire body needs to be focused on during a session and if you skip over any are the client will not receive all of the benefits they could from Reiki. If the client requests that you skip these areas make sure they understand they are missing out on some of the benefits of Reiki.

To get a lot of experience, offer to volunteer your services at a local hospital or nursing home. You will be bettering your skills while helping others as well.

Don't focus on charging a fee for Reiki sessions when you first start out. It is much more important that you focus on getting the experience that you need.

Continue with Reiki education. There are three levels of Reiki practitioners, one, two and three. The final level is a Reiki Master. There are courses you can take to move up in the levels and learn more and more about Reiki. As you move up in the levels you will be able to help more people. It is best to go to a Reiki Master for complete training. You can of course go to someone on one of the other levels but they will not be able to get you to a master level. Deciding how far you want to go though is completely up to you.

You can also create a personal Reiki box. To do this you will take a crystal and put it in a box with a lid, you will draw Reiki symbols on the inside of the box and place your intentions inside. You can place anything from becoming more productive to healing of heart disease to getting a specific amount of money. It is basically using Reiki, just as you would positive affirmations. You will do Reiki over the box for five minutes and from that moment on the box is activated. You can check your intentions once a week and tear up the ones that have been accomplished. You can also burn them releasing them to the universe.

A Reiki notebook can also be created. Again you will draw the Reiki symbols, and do a five minute Reiki over the notebook once this is complete the notebook is activated and you can write your requests in it.

Share the Reiki box or notebook with clients, family and friends. It will make your job much easier when they are in a session with you.

I stated earlier that you could work with a Reiki Master in order to fully learn Reiki but this is not necessary. Reiki is so simple and so safe that even a child can learn it. The great thing is that today many masters are posting videos online for those who want to learn. Once you learn, make sure to share your knowledge with others. As long as we continue to share Reiki, Reiki will continue.

When you begin Reiki, focus on self-healing, use your Reiki box or notebook for only yourself, focus on learning as much as you can about self-healing and once you have mastered that move on to helping others. Take the time you need to master each level and don't try to rush yourself because you want to do more this will only cause you to become frustrated and your Reiki will diminish.

Chapter 15: What Is Reiki?

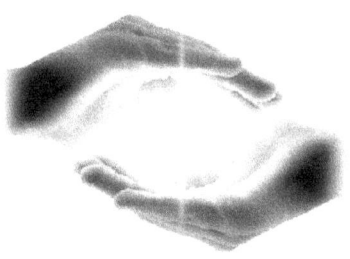

The practice of Reiki is of Japanese origin. The name is a combination of two Japanese words, Rei and Ki. While the translation can become a bit complicated, Rei is loosely related to the knowledge and energy that flows through everything. It is omniscient and knows all. It is often related to the idea of God in many religions. Ki, in simple terms, is the life force that rules the universe. When this Ki is high, we feel energetic and happy, and when it is low, we feel drained and ill.

The practice of Reiki harnesses the capabilities of both the Rei and Ki energy for healing. To practice Reiki, there must be a receiver and a practitioner. The receiver is the person in need of healing, whether it be a physical ailment, chronic disease or emotional state. The practitioner is in charge of focusing the energy of the universe into the receiver so that they may heal themselves.

A Reiki session is very relaxed and soothing. The practitioner takes their time, slowly connecting the palms of their hands with various points, usually in relation to chakras, on your body. This is not like a massage, as muscles are not being rubbed. The idea is simply to transfer energy from the practitioner to the receiver. This is done by simply holding the hands on the touch-point for a moderate length of time, before moving on to another point.

A practitioner does not hold the energy, only has the ability to draw it to the receiving person. Once a part of this person's energy field, it will go where it is needed most, at the site of the ailment. It is Ki that naturally energizes all vital organs, tissues, and cells. Without it, we develop serious illness and dysfunction within the body. Drawing in Ki from outside the body helps set the balance back in motion so that the body may do what it is supposed to do.

Unlike traditional Western medicine, this type of energy healing can do no harm, as the power to yield results is with the power of the universe. In modern medicine, fate is given to the hands of people, who often make mistakes. They give medications that do more harm than good. They carry out procedures that break the rules of nature. All in hopes of doing good, but actually disrupts the natural energy flow in the body, among many other things.

There is great control in the energy given by the universe. In fact, a person who is unwilling or skeptical about the practice rarely reaps the benefits. Positive energy from the universe can be upset by negative thoughts and emotions running through the body. Before getting started with any Reiki session, it is important to enter a relaxed state through meditation, so that energy will be allowed to flow freely throughout the body.

What is worse, it is this negative energy that is the likely cause of physical and emotional problems in the first place, making it extremely important to get our negative thoughts under control. The energy we are made up of is not contained within just the confines of our body. We actually have an energy field called an aura surrounding our bodies. We emanate energy.

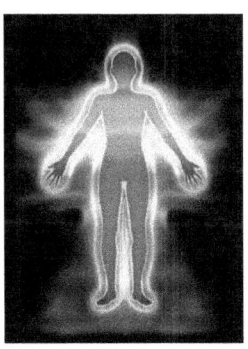

Certain people are very tapped into energy fields, and can actually recognize auras around themselves and others. Auras appear as light, often colored, which reflects the current emotional state of the person. Calm, relaxed blues and greens signify calm, while reds may denote anger in the aura. The color and strength of the aura can change at any given time based on your emotional and physical well-being. Auras are not one solid color or strength, it will vary. Think of it like the earth's ozone layer. Where the sun beats through, the ozone layer is thin, letting in more damaging solar rays. If your aura is thin in a specific area, there will likely be something physically wrong underneath. For example, if your aura is thin and red over your kidney region, it means that energy is restricted in this area and your kidney function could decline. Working on the aura in this region, as well as your chakra system will help bring energy back to the area, where it needs it most. As medical procedures become more common, we must ask ourselves what is really right for our bodies. Is it best to suppress symptoms of physical and mental ailments with medications and procedures, or is it better to unmask the problem behind the symptoms that will ultimately lead to a better quality of life?

As modern medicine advances, procedures are becoming less invasive, yet overall health is still on the decline. This begs us to find an alternative to these ways and getting back to the basic elements that make us up for answers.

While it is possible to attract positive energy to yourself, Reiki is most effective with a practiced healer, someone who is familiar with energy fields and has the ability to attract the most positive energy toward you. Remember that if your aura is weak, it will be hard to gather the strength to ask the universe for what you need. Don't be afraid to meet with a professional and give Reiki a try. Keep a positive, open mind going into the experience, and you won't regret it.

The benefit of Reiki is that it can help flush out the negative emotions and thoughts we have in our minds. Remember that positive energy is drawn to negative energy, and it will flow where it is needed most. The negativity may inhibit just how much energy we can accept, but it will work just the same. Having treatment frequently will help break down as much negativity as possible, eventually filling you with positivity.

Reiki is a very personal, unexplainable practice. If you have not had the pleasure of a Reiki session with a practiced Reiki master, it is highly recommended. We cannot truly explain in words the feeling of energy flowing through you, as this is a transcendental experience that will likely be different for each individual. You owe it to your inner spirit to try Reiki and find out the benefits for yourself.

Chapter 16: Benefits And Limitations Of Reiki

Reiki is a powerful resource, as you have already learned and been shown, as well as a unique way to understand the human body-mind-spirit connection and the experience of being a human being on more than one level. We are all available to use Reiki whenever we are ready to know what it can do for us and not all people are as interested or excited in the applications of what it is and how it works. As we continue to evolve as a species, we are showing new signs of growing interest in using these models and structures for healing as technology has made it possible for these types of information to be shared as easily as finding a grain of sand on a beach. There are people who have been utilizing the Reiki healing treatment methods for decades and as we slowly embrace a different process for resolving problems, we become more acquainted with the benefits, as well as all of the limitations of what a healing tool like Reiki offers.

The planet is shared by all people and we all have a responsibility to learn new ways to allow ourselves to evolve and change what is no longer serving us as a whole. There will always be long-term cycles of evolutionary technological advancement, or belief systems working hard to establish order, and even within the midst of all of that, one thing is ever the same: Universal Life Force.

The practice of Reiki includes all systems of the human body (emotional, spiritual, mental, physical) and works to help the consciousness evolve to accept our abilities to see each other from, and on, all of these levels without much effort or difficulty. The process is slow and it can take months or years of hard work, opening, and energetic shift in order for anything, or anyone to heal, and so as you look at the benefits and limitations of Reiki, you can understand why some of these things have slowed us down from accessing this energetic positivity more than we have as a world group.

The Benefits of Reiki

There are so many benefits to using Reiki as a healing method, you could write an entirely separate book about all of them. The reason is because Reiki isn't specific to only one type of issue or dysfunction. Reiki is always available and it assumes whatever position it needs to in the healing of energy surrounding all issues, whether they are major or minor.

The benefits of Reiki include all four systems of the human experience and so let's take a look at them on separate levels to paint a clearer picture:

Physical Benefits

Overall and general relaxed state in the body

Relief of pain

Long-term healing of scar tissue and deep wounds from surgical procedures

Regression of some illnesses and diseases, when used with other medical advice

Relief from chronic headache or migraine

Elimination of soreness, aches and pains

Progress in healing form the results of cancer treatments

Healthy results from working with AIDS and HIV, prolonging life and sometimes sustaining it in healthy ways

Broad spectrum healing of significant, or chronic problems with the ligaments, muscle fibers, and tissues

Helps balance blood sugar levels, and can help with some cases of diabetes (consult with your Reiki practitioner first)

Relief of joint pain and inflammation

Helps with sleep regulation

And more!

Mental Benefits

Processing of thoughts in a clearer way

Improvement of memory and cognitive function

Opening of clairvoyance and psychic potential

Shifting of old, outdated thought programs that keep you in low vibration or negativity

Promoting the healing possibilities with depression, paranoia, anxiety, etc.

Increasing state of calm, peace of mind and serenity

Invites opening to see beyond the parts of you that get trapped in thought cycles that are destructive

Helps remove habitual thought forms that create negative habits and thought patterns

Gives opening to heal the mind from false attitudes, belief systems or structures that are not a part of your true self

Can assist with helping people with neurodegenerative disorders

And more!

Emotional Benefits

Processing of emotional stagnation from old wounds and insecurities

Purging of repressed emotions or memories blocking healthy energetic flow

Safe and healthy emotional release, such as crying, sobbing, hysterical laughter

Difficult emotional bonds and links to other people resolved and processed

Feelings of joy and bliss

Creativity and expressiveness restored or opened wider

Passions ignited

Self-confidence, self-worth, self-esteem enhanced

Emotional agility expanded

Feelings of loss, pain and grief resolved

And more!

Spiritual Benefits

Spiritual awakening experiences, or ignition of Kundalini awakening

Opening of the Universal consciousness

Reverence for all things and all beings on the planet

Presence of psychic awareness and opening

Feelings of limitlessness

Ascension of the soul and journey into a higher vibrational frequency to become more "light"

Dramatic purging of limiting belief systems to allow for higher vibrational existence

Full chakra alignment to allow for oneness, wholeness and balance with the self and all life around you

And more!

As you can see, Reiki has quite a lot of benefit, and that wasn't even the whole list of possibilities. There are plenty of other ways, not listed here that can show you how powerful Reiki truly is. Here are some of the additional benefits of Reiki:

Useful in living spaces, dwellings, offices and other environments that require regular energy clearing, protection, or vibrational healing

Beneficial to plants and landscapes for growth and healing purposes, even in the home garden or potted plants

Helpful with aiding in the relaxation and calmness of children and infants

Excellent resource for prolonging the life of pets and keeping them in good health

Protection against mishaps during travel

And more!

Reiki is an excellent resource for healing and it isn't magic! It is a simple techniques and tool to harness the flow of high vibrational energy through the conduit of the self to help you and others heal. You are in good hands when you are in the hands of Reiki!

Almost all things have another side to them and nothing is perfect. The results of

Reiki can be incredibly challenging and difficult as it can create a lot of emotional upheaval, especially if you are not prepared to go through some changes. The next section will talk more about Reiki and how it can also have some limitations.

The Limitations of Reiki

Limitations don't always mean that they are negative or bad. Limitation can simply refer to the element or need to be aware of what can be challenging or difficult, especially when you are going through a healing journey. Most healing journeys have several ups and downs and as with anything, Reiki is an intense resurrection of thoughts, feelings, ideas, memories and past wounds and traumas that can really shake a person up.

The best way to interpret this is to show you how to heal from these moments and intentionally resolve some of these problems that arise, and as you look at some of these limitations, know that Reiki is a supportive tool to help you finally release and let go some of these side-effects and what might be considered limitations when brought up in your normal, everyday life.

Limitations and Challenges of Reiki

Opening and Releasing Past Hurts, Wounds and Traumas:

Resurrecting old wounds to purge and release them can cause a lot of pain to return to your mind and feelings. When we are hurt by something, we aren't always given the tools to process our feelings about them and so we stuff them down, hide them away and make them a part of our identity. Reiki burns through the hidden layers and calls the wounds to come up and out to help you resolve and release them for good. This emotional release can actually take weeks, and might involve other therapies to help you process your feelings from this kind of energetic release.

Healing from old hurts and pain can be very time consuming which is part of why many people will avoid digging up old traumas and learning to look at them so that they can be healed.

Trauma is debilitating and can even cause a return of the initial shock or PTSD that occurred in the original moment of trauma. This has to be handled with great care and can cause a lot of problems for someone who might have to go through a deeper process of healing. This can be limiting to the person if they are not in a mental or emotional position to handle that release and healing.

Life Changing Events Caused by Energetic Shift:

Reiki assumes a position of perfect knowledge of where to work, how long, and in what ways to heal, in order to truly bring you into a total ascension of self so that you are in your highest vibration. This can be life changing and can cause a lot of personal and professional drama.

You may be inclined to change your profession, career, lifestyle, diet, home, relationships and partnerships and so forth. So large life changes are not always possible at the drop of the hat and there can be challenges with how Reiki exposes you to this reality and asks you to embrace your wholeness and your truth.

There are no laws or rules about how you are going to feel after you go through a Reiki healing process and what you choose to do, so you may have a lot of emotional pain and drama, as well as difficult thoughts and feelings about how you are changing, which can effect your general happiness and overall outlook on life.

Reiki Isn't a Cure:

Many people want one magical thing to fix their pain and suffering, or a miracle drug or surgery to make them feel better, and this actually isn't how life works. Reiki can only help to provide support and energetically shift and heal you if you are willing to go on a long, deep, and beautiful journey of hard work and awakening.

There will always be situations that Reiki can only help, but not ultimately cure or completely eradicate. The balance of life and death, or light and dark is always present with Reiki and the symbols that you use in a healing treatment, but you cannot change the reality of certain outcomes.

Practicing Reiki on others is an amazing benefit to many people, but you can't fix every person and as a practitioner, you have to honor your limits and boundaries with allowing Reiki to be the Master and let yourself off the hook if you can't resolve someone's pain and suffering.

Reiki is an amazingly beneficial tool to use to inspire healing, change, growth, light and love, from within the self, and through all people who are opening to its possibilities. As with anything, nothing is perfect and all matters dealing with the human experience will be fraught with ups and downs, difficulties and challenges and beautiful opportunities for growth and expansion.

The only limit is the imagination, as far as what you can do with Reiki, and so if you are open to what it can offer, you also have to be open and honest with the results and that they can be challenging and not with out some limitations. Balance is the key with Reiki. In the next chapter, you will learn the power of the Reiki symbols and how they are used to enhance specific kinds of healing on all the levels discussed in this chapter.

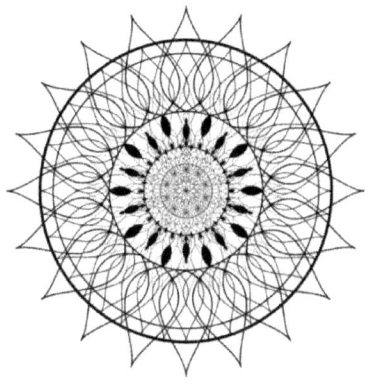

Chapter 17: Tools For Testing Your Energy

There are several ways that you can begin to work with Reiki on your own at home, with or without your first level attunement. It helps to have the instruction and attunement from the Reiki Master of your choosing, but you can also begin to explore self-healing methods by working with your own energy. It may take a lot of practice and energy at first, but you can begin to learn the subtle ways that your energy can shift if you follow these simple instructions.

This chapter will give you a few meditations, and some helpful instructions for connecting to your Reiki flow of energy. Remember that you are just a channel for this energy to pass through you; you are not the one healing- Reiki is. Reiki is the Universal life-force energy that can be channeled through your body and spirit to help you find the right path for healing.

The following tools will be best performed in a comfortable setting where you won't be disturbed and can focus and concentrate on your energy. If you have not already been attuned to Reiki, the following exercises can help you open your energy and connect with it more effectively so that you can feel it in your hands and the crown of your head.

Open Channels Exercise

Sitting comfortably on the floor or in a chair, keep your back straight and your eyes closed. If you need any additional supports for your body, you can prepare them now. You want to begin from a comfortable position so that you can focus on the energy and not on any difficult or uncomfortable body postures.

Focus on your breath and take several inhales and exhales in slow, deep counts.

Try to connect to yourself and let go of nagging thoughts, checklists, or anxiety about what's happening outside of you.

Breath in and out and release tension in your body. Find any areas that feel tight or tense and breathe out the stiffness.

When you are ready, place your hands on your knees, palms up.

Feel the centers of both palms. Feel the energy of these areas for a few moments. Try to focus and concentrate on any sensations of throbbing, buzzing, tingling, anything at all.

Now, focus your attention on the crown of your head. Feel the energy of this area. Keep your body still and relaxed with your palms still facing up, and notice any feeling in the crown of your head. Spend several minutes in this posture.

After you have engaged with these areas of focus, you can begin to visualize in your mind's eye, a white beam of light coming from up high and going straight through the top of your head and into your body.

Allow all of this light energy to fill your body. Notice if your energy changes at all when this light starts to come through you. Invite it in and offer your gratitude. If you feel compelled, you can lift your hands and perform a gassho, one of the pillars of Reiki. Give thanks for the Reiki energy coming through you.

Return your hands to your knees, palms up and begin to see the light pumping into the crown of your head and through your body coming out of the palm of your hands.

As the light beams out of your hands, pick your hands up and face them together, palm to palm, but do not touch them.

Get them as close as you can without touching. You may choose to open your eyes for this but try to keep them closed and just feel the energy.

As your hands come closer together, see if you can feel the energy field between your palms when they are not touching.

If you can feel anything then you are working with your Reiki energy channels being open through your palm chakras.

Begin to slowly move one hand in small circles with the palms still facing each other, like you are drawing a circle on the palm that is standing still. Your palms should not be touching and they should both be flat.

Continue to see the light coming through the crown of your head and your palms. Make sure you are still breathing deeply and slowly as you sense your palm energy.

This activity can last as long as you want it to. Play around with the palm circles and see if you can notice any changes in your feeling. Is it getting stronger? Is it magnetic, pulling your hands closer, or pushing them farther apart? Is there any tingling or humming sensation in your hands? Does it feel itchy?

Explore your energy. The point is to connect to your ability to be a direct channel of healing light.

Practice this exercise daily to help you improve your energy-sensing skills.

The next Reiki exercise will build upon this one so that you can take it to the next level. Let yourself be guided to what feels best for you while working with your energy. If you start to feel fatigued, light-headed, headachy, or any other discomfort, stop and relax, drink a glass of water and try eating a snack before going any further.

Moving Energy Exercise

This exercise is designed to help you connect with your auras and chakras a little bit more deeply. This can be a little harder if you are not yet attuned to Reiki by a Master, but you are still always affecting your energy, even if you are not feeling the movement of energy very strongly. You will learn more meditations to help you with this in Chapter 9, and this exercise tool will simply help you engage with your auras and chakras a little bit better.

To begin this exercise, start with the previous exercise you learned to get you warmed up. Spend 10-15 minutes warming up your hand chakras with the Open Channels exercise.

Once your channels are open, continue sitting, or lie down on a mat or other comfortable surface. You can perform this exercise sitting or lying down.

Adjust your body to feel comfortable and begin by placing your hands in a Mu-Shin gassho (hands, palm to palm, close to the heart, fingers pointed up to the chin).

Offer your gratitude and thanks to being a channel of light and love.

Separate your hands and begin to hold them so that your palms are facing your body. Let yourself be guided as much as possible in which direction they travel around your body.

You can hover your hands about 4 to 5 inches away from the body, or bring them closer if you feel the need. You don't have to touch your body for this to work.

Feel your energy by trying to move it around. Can you feel any changes in your palm chakras when you are moving over your heart versus over your crown? Do you feel any temperature changes when you are moving from one part of your body to the next?

Spend some quality time looking for movement or change in how your energy feels from one part of your body to the next. You can bring your attention to your chakras one by one and try to feel each one from the root to the crown, moving the Reiki energy with you through your palms as you go.

This tool is an exercise to help you become better acquainted with how Reiki will feel as you move energy through you. You are a channel for Reiki to pass through and the idea is that you allow it to guide you where you need to go. Surrendering this energy can be challenging at first, especially if you are not yet attuned to Reiki energy by a Master. Consider finding someone in your local area to help you shift your energy to Reiki level one or two to help you become a more open channel. Some Reiki Masters will even offer that process through a distance healing workshop that you can do online.

The more open your channels are, the easier it is for you to feel that energy coming through your crown, out of your hands and into your auras and chakras. The best practices are to keep going through both of these simple exercise tools daily until you feel a major shift in your energy. You can begin to feel your own energy more deeply the more you practice.

The next set of tools is to help you understand how to let yourself heal through these simple instructions. You may find it to be too simple and easy at first, but once you get through it and really explore yourself with it, you will understand just how truly impactful this Reiki tool really is.

Visualizing the Reiki Field

Reiki energy expresses itself in a lot of ways. For some people, it is a physical feeling where they feel energy only in the palms of the hands and perhaps in the crown of the head. At other times, there are very elaborate and creative visual experiences that help you better see the source of the trauma or wound you are healing through a specific description of it in the mind's eye.

You have certainly dreamed before and as such are familiar with how surreal the subconscious can be. Your mind uses the dreams state as a tool to help you unravel your experiences in a unique and creative way. Creative visualization works in the same way. When you are connected to a

Reiki channel, you are being shown through your third eye what needs to be healed and what you are working with. The images that come to you could manifest in a variety of ways and a lot of them may feel strange and unusual but for many doing this type of energy work, it is just part of the experience.

Accepting that you are a person who is capable of seeing your own wounds is a part of the practice of Reiki. If you get involved with helping other people, these visions will support their healing experiences. The main thing to note is that you not question what is happen and allow yourself to witness whatever imagery comes into your mind.

The power of the third eye is strong in all of us and for many people, this area can be blocked. This exercise can actually help you balance and open your third eye more effectively and once you are open in this chakra, you will be even more capable of channeling Reiki energy for self-healing purposes.

To begin, warm yourself up with the previous exercises, **Open Channels Exercise** and **Moving Energy Exercise**. You can spend about 15 minutes on those warm-ups before moving into these steps.

Perform a Mu-shin Gassho and recite the 5 principles of Reiki to yourself in your mind. Give yourself permission to be an open channel for Reiki and ask to be guided in your experience.

With your hands on your knees, face-up, allow Reiki energy to flow out of your palms. When you are seeing that energy in your third eye, you are ready to begin your Visualization exercise.

Allow yourself to be guided to the area that needs healing. Let yourself naturally go there. Release any ideas you have and surrender to the energy of Reiki.

Bring your focus and attention to the area you have been guided to and in your head, ask Reiki to show you what needs to be healed. Offer your gratitude for being shown the right path for healing.

Give your mind plenty of time to recognize what you are seeing. Anything could come up, an old memory, a picture of a person, a boat floating on the sea, a hot air balloon in a stormy sky. You could also see shadowy objects in your auric field, that look like dark shards, stones, or crystals. Try not to guess and just allow yourself to see whatever image rises to the surface.

Whatever you end up seeing in your auras or chakras is what you are dealing with in the Reiki field. Reiki is showing you an idea or an image of how to heal a certain area. It could be as intricate as a well-known landscape from your childhood memories, or as simple as a colorful pool of water that looks like a wheel of light energy.

Try not to force anything about it and just let yourself look. The Reiki field is asking you to see what it wants to show you. You are not going to show it what it should be doing. Reiki is how you learn to let go of your mind's control over what is so that you can truly see.

Give some time and space to let these visions come and spend time just witnessing your energy. Try not to influence the outcome of the visions you are receiving and let the Reiki field just show you how to heal your energy.

Practice with this cycle of visualizing as often as you can until it feels easy to achieve.

A visualization is a tool of Reiki. It is part of what helps you see the Reiki field and what lies beyond the understanding of the mind so that you can see the spirit. You are always able to see this part of yourself and we are just not taught to look at ourselves in this way, through this landscape of reality. It is just as real as what you can see with your physical eyes.

The tool of visualization will help you connect better to how you will be healing your own energy, showing you the map and blueprint of what path you should be taking right now. You don't need to be attuned to Reiki to practice this type of visualization tool, but you will be able to get more out of the experience if you are attuned by a Master.

These three exercises are some of the best tools you can use to begin working with Reiki and enjoying it in your everyday life.

You don't have to be attuned or an expert to begin self-healing with Reiki. All you need is a little practice, a lot of focus, and an urge to dig more deeply into your energy fields with Reiki as your guide.

Chapter 18: Universal Radiation, Understanding The Aura

Do you know why Christmas is always a magical experience for kids? It is because of the continuing tradition with Christmas gifts, Santa Clause, holiday cheer, and every other thing that makes the season special. So, a child goes through this process from a tender age till he or she becomes a teenager and will always remember the magic of Christmas.

Now, Reiki isn't a seasonal experience like Christmas, but it can completely transform your life in a wholesome way. So, why not think about sustaining this feeling?

Some people discover the excitement of Reiki, bask in the feeling for a few days, and forget about the experience. Others, however, do not forget intentionally but say, "Life happens." This is why they must take an intentional approach towards ensuring that they sustain and continue the healing process.

More often than not, when there is a discourse on universal energy and treatment options, there is very little attention to how people can sustain what they learn and keep up with their sessions.

Nothing good will last long if there is no effort to ensure its continuity. You want to make sure that this fantastic experience you have going for yourself continues and that you are inspired to do more with Reiki other than simply know how it works.

This chapter will introduce you to some ideas that will ensure the continuity of your Reiki experience. It is the perfect way to bring this journey to an end.

Note: The steps you will find below cut across what both healers and recipients can do to sustain the practice. So, depending on what you are going after, there is an idea for both sides of the treatment option.

How to Sustain Reiki in Your life

Show Up for Sessions

If you are very serious about sustainability with your Reiki practice and healing, then you must develop the discipline to show up for all your recommended meetings. There is a small group of people who believe that Reiki doesn't work and that it isn't as effective as the healers make it be. Such people speak from the incompetent experiences they had and will do whatever they can to make others believe them.

Well, the reason why they say that is because they didn't complete their sessions or stick to the advice or caution of the practitioners. While others have amazing Reiki stories to tell, they don't. If you don't show up for sessions, you will end up like such person.

It takes a lot of commitment to get the best out of Reiki. In some situations, one session is enough. For others, though, you will need more than one. Still, the decision isn't yours to make, especially if you aren't doing self-treatment. The healer will decide on that because he or she is the one who is handling the session and will know what you need.

If you aspire to become a professional healer someday, how do you intend to help your patients get better when you can't adhere to your own healer's advice? Reiki is never about convenience or a perfectly suited time or when you feel like doing it.

If you have a pressing challenge, and you are keen on taking care of it, you must be willing to do whatever is required to make it happen. We are not talking about achieving healing today and struggling with the same thing the next week; we are seeking ways through which you can become a walking testimony of the impact of Reiki and achieve that. Therefore, consistency with sessions is required.

Now I know that some individuals may have hectic schedules, even though they genuinely want to complete their sessions. If you are such a person, then you must learn how to prioritize and manage your time well enough so that you can do everything necessary.

Reiki practitioners are not just all about helping you with your ailment or psychological challenge. They are also humane individuals who are trained to understand the value of time. Instead of procrastinating your sessions or not showing up for them at all, reach out to your healer and explain your peculiar situation.

Let the healer know that you are willing to work around your schedule, but you need help. By doing this, you will be helping yourself as you take on so many things at once, which can lead to stress. Now, you want to ensure that you can sustain the Reiki impact. If you don't know how to manage it with your schedule, speak to your healer.

It wouldn't be nice if, after reading this book, you end up like some people who say that Reiki doesn't work because you didn't commit to the process entirely. We have not only been on a journey together with this book, but you have also invested in your life by purchasing it. So, how do you get the dividends of the investment?

You achieve the latter by being committed to the process and ensuring that you give it your best at all times. You can sustain the Reiki impact. Start by not missing out on sessions, and you will be amazed at the level of progress you make with your experience long-term.

Be Attentive to Your Body

Another step that you can take towards sustaining Reiki is being attentive to your body. Reiki is all about energy, and energy is about awareness. In fact, if you are not someone who is easily attuned or discerning of energy around yourself, you surely cannot get the benefits of Reiki long-term. Meaning, if you are not someone who pays close attention to these things, you will need more practice, and the best way to do that is by listening to your body.

Your body speaks to you all the time. The question is, are you listening? Are you paying attention to the signs and signals that it's sending to you? Some people go for a Reiki session; because they are not attentive to their bodies, though, they don't know what takes place in it. They don't know if they have been healed; they cannot feel the energy permeate their bodies. For this reason, they can never succeed with the idea of sustainability as well.

After ensuring that you have not skipped even one session, you should pay close attention to what your body is trying to say to you. That is the only way you can ascertain the extent of healing you've received and anything else.

Below, you will discover a step that advises you to share your experience with others and help them, but how do you intend sharing with them when you don't know what happened to you? When you are sharing your story with people, and they ask questions regarding the impact of Reiki on your body, what will you say? If you haven't been listening to your body, today is an excellent time to start.

Shut out the noise around you for a few minutes every day. Some people call it meditation, but this time you will seek to listen to your voice. When you shut out everything, wait for a few minutes. With your mind's eye, roam around your body and listen to your heartbeat. Does it seem regular to you? Do you feel tired? Is your body saying something through your new sleep duration?

I am so keen on helping you listen to your body because a lot of ailments and problems that people seek Reiki for are preventable if they have paid attention to their bodies. So, in those moments when you listen, if there is something amiss, share it with your healer or practice Reiki on yourself using the hand movements you've been taught earlier.

Over time, you will find that you don't need to run to the hospital every time there is a little health scare because your body communicates with you, and you listen to it. The universal energy that you get through Reiki will also keep your body stable, so you are always healthy, optimistic, and excited about life.

Learn More

It doesn't matter what you think you already know. There is always more to learn, especially if you want to be a Reiki healer or practitioner for a long while. The most successful therapists do not stop learning. In fact, they intentionally study every day because they realize that nothing will stay the same all year long.

If you don't make attempts to learn and discover more about Reiki, you will become obsolete. Hence, you will no longer be as effective as you used to be. As recipients feel like they are not getting help from you, they will seek other Reiki healers, and you will lose clients.

Building a good reputation as a healer is part of the process. You don't become a reputable one all of a sudden. It takes a lot of work, which lies within your ability to make the sessions work.

Don't stop learning Reiki with this book. Read more materials, listen to successful practitioners, attend seminars and workshops, register for personal coaching lessons, and even do some on-the-job training to know what it's like to work with recipients. If you are committed to the idea of sustainability, then it means you want to practice for a long time. For that to happen, you must be committed to continuing and vigorously learning new procedures.

Think about doctors, lawyers, and people in other professions. It takes them quite a while to become professionals; they go through years of training at varying levels of difficulty as well. You are dealing with the idea that will liberate a lot of individuals from their challenges, and you are attuned to the universe. For this reason, you must take your profession seriously as well.

In the olden days when Reiki just became popular, it wasn't so easy for people who desired to become healers to get further training. Some even had to travel to learn from masters. These days, though, technology has made it easier for anyone who is willing to gain knowledge about Reiki.

Meanwhile, if you don't have money to pay for the more exclusive trainings, you can start with the free ones from blogs. There are also online platforms that are solely dedicated to Reiki training. Before adopting any of the approaches you see virtually, make sure that the website is verified and that you are getting authentic content that suits your desire for success with Reiki.

The more you learn and practice, the better you become, and then you can advance to higher heights with your Reiki practice. You wouldn't learn everything within a specified time frame, so I cannot tell you that it will take one or two years. Several doctors with years of experience still get to learn new facts about their profession every day, after all. If you are keen on being the best in this field, therefore, you must be willing to become aggressive and committed to learning.

Don't Be Selfish

This step is so important, and we cannot bring this book to a close without talking about it. If you are practicing or intend to practice Reiki selfishly with the sole aim of making money, you will be causing a lot of harm to your reputation and the field in general.

Do not practice Reiki just because you want to profit from clients or gain control and prestige. You will have a stubborn time proving your expertise if you do that.

Also, Reiki isn't about you, your selfish motives, or what you will derive from it.

Reiki is all about the person who is healed, as well as the role of the healer in connecting the life force energy to the recipient. What's most striking is the fact that you will not be able to establish a thriving practice because you would struggle with gaining access to guidance from the spirit.

If your connection to the universal energy doesn't have a strong spiritual base, then you cannot tap into the universe's energy quickly. A motive is significant since, as a healer, you will be the conduit for the healing the recipient will receive. What kind of channel you want to be, a selfish one who only thinks about themselves? Alternatively, do you want to become a selfless channel?

You must get to know what your motives are before taking the next step towards practicing Reiki. Don't decide on becoming an expert because it seems like a good title or business idea. You must look beyond yourself and what you will gain and continually strive to seek the greater good of all men and women who may cross your path.

If you have read through this book, and you feel that stirring sensation within you to make a difference in the world, then it means that Reiki is for you. When you pursue it, you can be sure of gaining success in this field. On the contrary, if all you see is a business opportunity, I will advise you not to take any step further towards becoming a Reiki practitioner now.

Spread the Word, Help Others

Sustainability will not be possible without the people who want to try out Reiki. So, if you are not concerned about anyone else but yourself, why are you reading this book? It is essential for everyone who wants to practice Reiki, as well as the ones who benefit from it, to take a step forward by reaching out to others.

Think about this for a second. If the earliest practitioners didn't try to help other people, would we ever know about Reiki today? You see, this step has been in use for years now because it is the one thing that guarantees sustainability.

This book and several others in this niche were written by seasoned authors who want to contribute their know-how to the sustainability movement by keeping the topic alive within most human interactions. Hence, if you have a successful Reiki story, why aren't you sharing it?

People only believe what they know can happen. We trust medicines, hospitals, and doctors because we have been taking drugs since we were kids and getting cured of illnesses. However, imagine if a doctor comes forward and says something can work, but he or she doesn't have any proof. Will you believe this physician and take a chance?

Theoretical knowledge doesn't inspire people. After all, anyone can write anything they want. Nevertheless, when individuals hear your distinct story when they know that this thing can transform their lives for good in ways they can only imagine, they will be willing to take a step towards it.

There are two ideas that are related to sustainability. The first one is the concept of spreading the word, and the second one is the concept of helping others. You cannot do one and leave the other. As you take steps towards spreading the word about Reiki, to be specific, you will have to reach out to help others as well.

Now, you don't have to take on an entire neighborhood or a bunch of people at the same time. Sart with your closest friends and family members who may be dealing with one health challenge or another. Introduce them to Reiki and then explain in detail what Reiki is about. If they have questions, try to provide answers but do not exaggerate anything so that they will not have to hold on to unrealistic expectations. If they are keen on books, you can share this book with them.

Considering your loved ones are excited about Reiki enough to want to give it a try, then you can use the second approach, which entails helping others. You try a

Reiki treatment session on them to help with their challenge. If you have been self-treating yourself, and you haven't healed someone else before, it may feel strange to you at first. Still, there's no need to worry because we know that you can do this!

Just ensure that you have practiced on yourself long enough and that you have achieved results before helping someone else. Doing self-treatment and treating others are the same. Only, with the latter, you will be channeling the universal energy into someone else's body.

Even if you have a friend who is far away, you can use the distant healing techniques you were taught earlier to make it happen. The point is that, by reaching out to others who need help, you will not only be contributing positively to someone else's life, but you will also be advancing your skills and getting better every day.

Take some time off to practice so that you can feel confident about what you are doing. Sustainability is all about carrying on with the tradition we gained (as others did before us). It is your contribution to the Reiki story. Although it may not be a story that is told globally, in your little way, you will be adding value to the lives of others.

There is more to say and achieve with Reiki, so take time to dig in through research. As you learn more, you will become empowered to share with the world what you have gained. Most healers are inspired by their desire to make the world a better place, to be honest. They see their gift not as a skill but as a medium through which they can contribute positively to the well-being of others.

Conclusion

Reiki is available to everyone, including children, the elderly, and the sick. We can all be a Reiki channel. There is no age limit, nor does it require any precondition. The technique training does not last long, and each level can be taught in one-day seminars. The technique is safe, without side effects or contraindications, being compatible with any other type of therapy or treatment. It is not a religious or philosophical system that proposes restrictions or taboos. It does not use talismans, prayers, visualizations, faith, or any object for its practical application. This technique is not obsolete; it remains the same for thousands of years.

After the energy tuning that occurs during the seminar, you can apply Reiki immediately for the rest of your life, even if you stop practicing it for a long period, and there is no need for a new activation for the same level. The energy is not polarized; it is neither positive nor negative (yin and yang).

www.ingramcontent.com/pod-product-compliance
Lightning Source LLC
Chambersburg PA
CBHW072009070526
44583CB00015B/1409